Paramedic Handbook

About the Author

Steven A. Jensen is a Colorado Certified Paramedic who graduated from the Swedish Medical Center's Program in 1977. He is currently practicing with the Weld County Ambulance Service and is a Mobile Intensive Care Paramedic (mission leader) for North Colorado Medical Center's Air Life helicopter transport team. He is also certified as a vocational instructor and an American College of Emergency Physicians Certified ACLS Provider.

Paramedic Handbook

by
Steven A. Jensen
EMT—Paramedic

Multi-Media Publishing, inc.
Denver, Colorado

Printed in the United States of America

MULTI—MEDIA PUBLISHING, INC., BOOK DIVISION
1393 S. INCA STREET, DENVER, COLORADO 80223

Library of Congress Cataloging in Publication Data

Jensen, Steven A., 1951—
Paramedic handbook.

Bibliography: p.
1. Medical emergencies—Handbooks, manuals, etc.
I. Title. [DNLM: 1. Emergency medical technicians.
2. Allied health personnel—Handbooks. 3. Emergencies—Handbooks. WX 215 J54p]
RC86.7.J46 1983 616'.025 82-42830

ISBN 0-940122-05-7 (pbk.)

MMP/B/B 9 8 7 6 5 4 3 2 1

Dedicated to:

— Doris Robertson, R.N., E.M.T., Instructor, Friend

— R. Adams Cowley, M.D., Maryland Institute for Emergency Medical Services, Shocktrauma Center, for his support of the paramedic system

— The patients served by the EMS System

PREFACE

The paramedic in the field has long needed a pocket review resource for emergency procedures and medications. While most emergency service personnel are constantly engaged in emergency care and continuing education, some may never treat or review the care of an injured diver; still others may see several such injuries a year, but they may never treat high altitude pulmonary edema. It is to provide a pocket emergency care resource that we have directed our efforts.

Please become familiar with the brief format and outline form employed in this handbook. Generally, signs and symptoms are given first, followed by treatment guidelines. A section for additional notes has been provided to allow inclusions or notations of changes.

NOTE: The treatment and care guidelines published here are just that—guidelines. They are not intended for use as protocols without the approval of a physician sponsor. They ARE intended to be a reminder of general care. Every effort has been made to ensure that both the treatments and drug information presented are accurate and in accord with accepted standards at the time of publication. Provisions have been made on each drug information page to enter dosages or uses that are unique to the user's area.

ACKNOWLEDGMENTS

This handbook is the result of special care and attention on the part of many persons. I would like to take this opportunity to thank especially the following:

— Editor David Spilver, for his support and belief in this project

— The EMS Divisions of:
- Swedish Medical Center, Englewood, CO
- Poudre Valley Hospital, Ft. Collins, CO
- North Colorado Medical Center, Greely, CO

for my educational experiences—practical, classroom and continuing

— Multi-Media Publishing, Inc., Denver, Colorado, for all the assistance and attention to detail

— Dr. Peter Bryson for his review of the drug section

— Dr. Frank Purdie for his review of the arrhythmias and treatments section

— Dr. Juan Nieto for the outline used in the treatment protocols

— Eunice Tokatloglou, R.N., for her review of the medical sections

Well done!
S.J.

Table of Contents

Part 4

Part 5

Part 6

Part 7

Introduction

This handbook is designed for use as a ready reference for emergency procedures and drug administration in the field. It is not intended to teach emergency care skills, rather it is intended to refresh the memory. The format of the book allows easy access to vital information.

Most procedures and drug dosages in the Handbook conform to DOT guidelines. Those procedures and dosages presented, but not found in DOT guidelines, are generally accepted standards that have found wide usage in the emergency care field.

Procedures are grouped within the text by the nature of the injury, illness or condition involved. Medications are presented alphabetically by generic name, following P.D.R. precedence.

The table of contents provides a page breakdown for each of the seven parts of PARAMEDIC HANDBOOK. The seven parts are also indexed by page-edge ink markings that allow easy location of each part. Additionally, each procedure or drug listing in the contents provides a specific page number for that individual listing to make location easier.

Entries are listed alphabetically within each part. Whether the reader refers to the table of contents or the title page for each part, subjects covered are easy to find.

Throughout PARAMEDIC HANDBOOK, space has been provided to allow individualization of information pertaining to procedure and drug administration protocols. Emergency service personnel will find the ability to note local variances and protocols especially helpful when facing unusual or infrequently encountered emergency situations.

Drug dosages presented within procedure discussions are the normal adult dosages for a specific situation. In Part 6, "Medications and Procedure Protocols," the standard dosages of a particular drug for both adult and pediatric patients are given. Throughout the handbook, when specific drugs are recommended, the reader is referred to detailed drug information in Part 6.

Charts and tables in PARAMEDIC HANDBOOK allow a clear, accurate understanding of conversions, dosages and procedural steps, and serve as quick field references.

Part 7 contains a list of emergency drugs and their classifications. Sections for emergency phone numbers, radio telemetry codes, and abbreviations and symbols used in field charting are also provided. A complete, step-by-step patient survey outline completes Part 7, "Field References."

Emergency service personnel who familiarize themselves with the format and features of PARAMEDIC HANDBOOK will find it to be an invaluable resource that can be easily carried and used in the field.

PART ONE
Cardiac and Related Problems

Arrhythmias and Treatments
Adult Arrest (Cor-Zero) Flow Chart
Cardiac Contusion
Cardiac Tamponade
Cardiogenic Shock
Chest Pain
Congestive Heart Failure
EKG Rate Table

Note:
Only normal adult dosages are provided here. See the drug section for pediatric dosages and more information.

SINUS ARRHYTHMIA

P	—	Normal, associated with QRS
QRS	—	Normal, less than .10 sec.
T	—	Normal
Rate	—	60 to 100
Rhythm	—	Irregular, changes with respiration
RX	—	None

SINUS TACHYCARDIA

P	—	Normal
QRS	—	Normal
T	—	Normal
Rate	—	Abnormal, 100 to 180
Rhythm	—	Regular

TREATMENT

- TREAT UNDERLYING CAUSES (pain, hypoxia, shock, fever, congestive failure, O.D.—including vasopressors, caffeine, isoproterinol, nicotine, aminophylline, and thyroid medications)
- Other ______________________________

____

ATRIAL FIBRILLATION

P	—	300 to 700 if present; irregular in rate and configuration
QRS	—	Usually normal, not preceded by a a demonstrable P wave. Aberrant conduction may distort the shape of the QRS.
T	—	Usually normal
Rate	—	160 to 180
Rhythm	—	Irregularly irregular, except in the digitalis intoxicated patient

continued

TREATMENT

- CARDIOVERSION IF COMATOSE OR HEMODYNAMICALLY UNSTABLE
  - 25J in previously digitalized patient; increase with caution
  - 50J and increase energy after each unsucessful defibrillation. Diazepam* may be indicated if the patient is conscious.
- DIGITALIZATION*
- QUINIDINE OR PROCAINAMIDE MAY CONVERT A PATIENT TO NSR.
- Other ______________________________

____

ATRIAL FIBRILLATION (with EKG indications of Digitalis Intoxication)

P, QRS and T are same as above and:
- High degree AV block (long R-R interval)
- Mobitz I AV block (decreasing R-R before a pause)
- 3° AV block with junctional (regular) rhythm
- PVC's

TREATMENT

- Withhold digoxin (see ATRIAL FIBRILLATION CAR—DIOVERSION)
- Other ______________________________

____

* *See drug section for use*

continued

ATRIAL FLUTTER

P — 240 to 360 sawtooth pattern (best seen in 2, 3, aVf)
QRS — Normal, often 2:1 conduction
T — Normal
Rate — 140 to 160
Rhythm — Regular

TREATMENT

- CARDIOVERSION IF HEMODYNAMICALLY UNSTABLE (start with 50J, unless the patient is on digoxin; then start with 25J.)
- DIGITALIZATION*
- Other ______________________________

____

SINUS BRADYCARDIA

P — Normal
QRS — Normal
T — Normal
Rate — Less than 60
Rhythm — Regular

TREATMENT

- HEMODYNAMICALLY UNSTABLE:
  - 0.5 atropine* q 5 min. to rate of 70 to 110 or Max 2mg. Isoproterinol* drip if there is no response to atropine.
- PACER
- Other ______________________________

____

SINUS ARREST

P — Normal, associated with QRS when SA node fires. (The entire P-QRS-T complex is skipped when the SA node does not fire.)
QRS — Normal
T — Normal
Rate — Normal to slow
Rhythm — Irregular when SA arrests

** See drug section for use*

continued

TREATMENT

- HEMODYNAMICALLY UNSTABLE:
  - 0.5 atropine* q 5 min. to rate of 70 to 110 or Max 2mg. Isoproterinol* drip, if indicated.
- Other ______________________________

____

PREMATURE ATRIAL CONTRACTIONS

P	—	Normal, except the P wave of the early beat has a different shape or may be hidden in the QRS
QRS	—	Normal or aberrantly conducted
T	—	Normal
Rate	—	Determined by number of PAC's
Rhythm	—	Irregular

TREATMENT

- None

PAROXYSMAL ATRIAL TACHYCARDIA

P	—	Normal or hidden
QRS	—	Normal
T	—	Normal or misshaped by P waves
Rate	—	150 to 220
Rhythm	—	Regular

TREATMENT

- VAGAL MANEUVERS, including MAST pants
- VERAPAMIL 0.075 to 0.15mg/kg (Max 10mg) over 10 min.
- EDROPHONIUM (TENSILON®) 1mg IV. After one min. without results, give 5 to 10mg over 30 to 60 sec.
- HEMODYNAMICALLY UNSTABLE: Cardioversion starting at 50J
- Other ______________________________

____

* *See drug section for use*

continued

PREMATURE JUNCTIONAL/NODAL CONTRACTIONS

- P — When present, differs from preceding or following P waves; P-R less than .12
- QRS — Normal, unless aberrant conduction present
- T — Normal or misshaped by P waves
- Rate — Determined by number of PJC's
- Rhythm — Regular to irregular

TREATMENT

- None

1° AV BLOCK

- P — P-R greater than .20
- QRS — Normal
- T — Normal
- Rate — 60 to 100 (may be seen in faster or slower rates)
- Rhythm — Regular

TREATMENT

- **None–MAY WARN OF IMPENDING 2° OR 3° BLOCKS**

2° AV BLOCK, MOBITZ I

- P — Normal, regular rhythm. P-R progressively lengthens until the QRS is dropped.
- QRS — Normal
- T — Normal
- Rate — Slow to normal
- Rhythm — Irregular due to block of impulse from SA

TREATMENT

- HEMODYNAMICALLY UNSTABLE: 0.5mg atropine* q 5 min. to rate of 70 to 110 or to Max 2mg. Isoproterinol drip, if indicated.
- PACER (Precordial or Pacemaker)
- Other ______________________

____

* *See drug section for use*

continued

373-5734

2° AV BLOCK, MOBITZ II

P — More P waves than QRS complexes (P-R may be greater than .20 sec.)
QRS — Normal, preceded by P wave (P to R ratio is 2:1, 3:1 . . .)
T — Normal
Rate — Normal to slow
Rhythm — Regular, unless variably blocked

TREATMENT

- AS FOR MOBITZ I

3° AV BLOCK

P — Normal, P-P regular 60 to 100
QRS — Occasionally normal, but usually aberrantly conducted
T — Normal
Rate — Nodal at 40 to 60 or idioventricular at less than 40
Rhythm — Usually regular

TREATMENT

- See Mobitz I
- Never give lidocaine.
- Other ______________________

____

PVC's

P — Not seen in association with QRS complex, unless PVC is interpolated
QRS — Distorted, wide (greater than .12 sec.)
T — Usually opposite of QRS

Note:
WATCH FOR PVC's IN NUMBERS GREATER THAN SIX PER MIN., MULTIFOCAL, R-ON-T, RUNS OR SALVOS, AND BIGEMINY.

continued

TREATMENT

- LIDOCAINE 1mg/kg FOLLOWED WITH A DRIP IF THERE IS NO INDICATION OF CONDUCTION DEFECTS, AND THE PATIENT IS HAVING CARDIAC PAIN.
- ATROPINE*, IF PVC's ARE RATE DEPENDENT
- Other ______________________________

____

VENTRICULAR TACHYCARDIA

EKG — Wide QRS complexes (greater than .12), cyclic, bizzare in shape, rate of 140 to 200 (looks like runs of PVC's)

TREATMENT

- STABLE:
  - LIDOCAINE* 1mg/kg FOLLOWED WITH A DRIP. BRETYLIUM* 5 TO 10mg/kg OVER 10 MIN.
- UNSTABLE:
  - CARDIOVERT: start at 25J; increase as needed. If the condition persists, give LIDOCAINE as above and repeat.
- AFTER CONVERSION:
  - LIDOCAINE OR BRETYLIUM DRIP (whichever caused conversion)
  - LIDOCAINE-BOLUS AND DRIP (if no medications were given)
- Other ______________________________

____

VENTRICULAR FIBRILLATION

EKG — Grossly irregular baseline without QRS or pulses

TREATMENT

- TWO MIN. OF EFFECTIVE CPR then defibrillate 400J (back-to-back, if first defibrillation was ineffective)
- If V-fibrillation still persists:
  - RECHECK CPR
  - SODIUM BICARBONATE* 1meq/kg
  - EPINEPHRINE* 0.5mg
  - DEFIBRILLATION (back-to-back)

* *See drug section for use*

continued

- LIDOCAINE* 1mg/kg
- DEFIBRILLATION
- BRETYLIUM* 5 to 10mg/kg

• After conversion:
  - LIDOCAINE OR BRETYLIUM DRIP (whichever caused conversion)
• Other ______________________________

ASYSTOLE

EKG — No cardiac activity; no pulses

TREATMENT

• SODIUM BICARBONATE* 1meq/kg; then half initial dose q 15 min.
• EPINEPHRINE* 0.5 to 1mg
• ATROPINE* 1 to 2mg
• CALCIUM CHLORIDE* 5cc of 10%
• REPEAT
• PRECORDIAL PACING
• PACEMAKER
• Other ______________________________

ELECTROMECHANICAL DISSOCIATION

EKG — Cardiac electrical activity without pulses

TREATMENT

• MAST* or fluid challenge may be ordered
• SODIUM BICARBONATE* 1meq/kg; then half initial dose q 15 min.
• EPINEPHRINE* 0.5 to 1mg
• CALCIUM CHLORIDE* 5cc of 10%
• ISOPROTERINOL* DRIP
• PRECORDIAL PACING
• CONSIDER PERICARDIOCENTESIS*
• Other ______________________________

* *See drug section for use*

ADULT ARREST (COR-ZERO) FLOW CHART

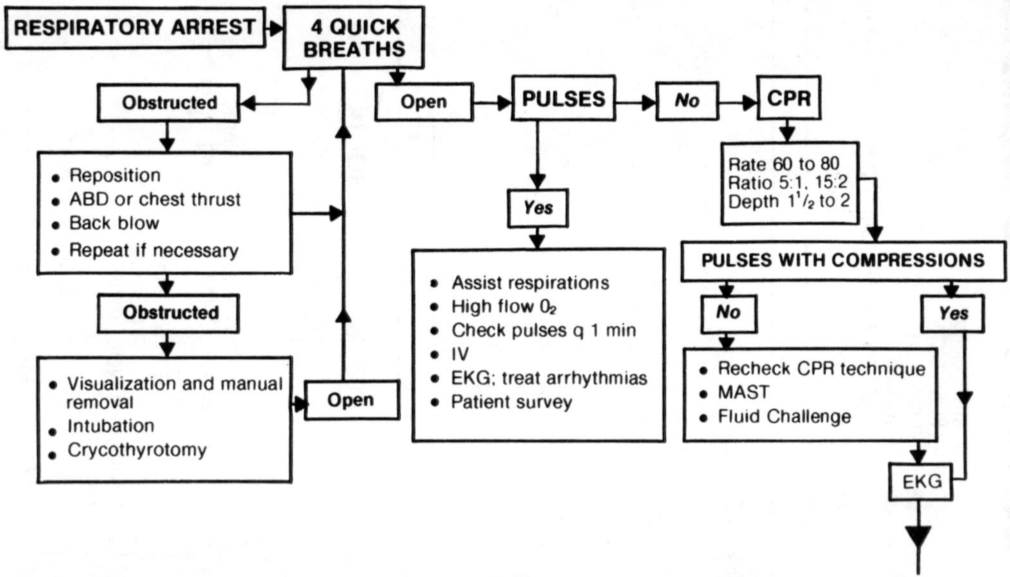

Asystole	Bradycardia	Electromechanical Dissociation	Ventricular Tachycardia	Ventricular Fibrillation
O_2	O_2	O_2	Cardioversion	Defib
IV	IV	IV	IV	Treat Arrhythmias
BICARB	BICARB	BICARB	LIDOCAINE	O_2
EPI	ATROPINE	Intubate	Treat Arrhythmias	IV
Intubate	Intubate	Fluid Challenge	O_2 and intubate	BICARB
ATROPINE	ISOPROTERINOL	EPI	BICARB	EPI
CALCIUM		CALCIUM		Defib
ISOPROTERINOL				LIDOCAINE
Defib				Defib

LIST YOUR DOSAGES HERE

ATROPINE ____________ EPINEPHRINE ____________ CARDIOVERT ____________

BICARBONATE ____________ ISOPROTERINOL ____________ DEFIBRILLATION ____________

CALCIUM ____________ LIDOCAINE ____________

✱ CARDIAC CONTUSION

SIGNS AND SYMPTOMS

1. Blunt trauma to the chest with or without fractured ribs
2. Chest pain
3. BBB on EKG
4. ST or T wave changes
5. Arrhythmias
   - Right-sided injury = Atrial Arrhythmias and RBBB
   - Left-sided injury and Frontal injury = Ventricular irritability

TREATMENT

- O_2
- IV D_5W TKO (to keep open)
- Monitor chest for developing signs of injury of compromise
- EKG (monitor closely as arrhythmias develop rapidly)
- Medications as indicated by arrhythmias

Note:

ACUTE PERICARDIAL TAMPONADE MAY DEVELOP

See Also:

Pneumothorax, tension pneumothorax, flail chest, pulmonary edema

CARDIAC TAMPONADE

SIGNS AND SYMPTOMS

1. Narrowing of pulse pressure
2. Decreasing Bp—initially elevated
3. Distended neck veins
4. Distant heart sounds progressively getting fainter
5. Shock syndrome
6. Pulsus alternans
   - Alternating weak and strong pulses may also be found in PAT, left ventricular failure, AV block or digitalis intoxication
7. Pulsus paradoxus (found in one-third of all tamponade)
   - Deflate Bp cuff until the first systolic sound is heard. Note this pressure. (Sound should disappear on inspiration.).
   - Continue deflation until all sounds are heard on inspiration and expiration.
   - A difference of 10mmHg is considered paradoxical.
8. Electrical alternans on EKG (alternating voltage height)
9. Cardiac rub (heard when patient sits forward)
10. Post cardiac surgery (may occur up to several months post-op)

TREATMENT

- O_2 Max
- IV
- ALS/CPR
- Isoproterinol* to enhance cardiac output
- Physician may order needle aspiration of pericardium or a fluid challenge

** See drug section for use*

CARDIOGENIC SHOCK

SIGNS AND SYMPTOMS

1. Bp less than 80
2. Tachycardia—normal
3. Shock syndrome
4. History of previous AMI/or current AMI
5. Arrhythmias
6. Patient taking digitalis
7. No evidence of blood loss
8. No response to fluid challenge
9. CHF
10. Heart murmer

TREATMENT

- O_2 and respiratory support as needed
- IV D_5W TKO (a fluid challenge may be ordered; MAST may be a reversible challenge)
- O_2 and intubation if comatose
- EKG
- Treat arrhythmias if this is the cause.
- Monitor vital signs and use vasopressors, if indicated.
- Sodium bicarbonate* may be ordered.
- Monitor for development of pulmonary edema.

See Also:
CHF

* *See drug section for use*

SIGNS AND SYMPTOMS

1. Sharp or crushing pain in chest (sometimes indigestion)
2. Radiating pain (to neck, jaw, arms, across chest)
3. Cool, diaphoretic skin
4. Pallor/cyanosis
5. Anxiety/restlessness
6. Hx of previous AMI
7. On cardiac medication
8. Irregular pulse
9. Check breath sounds
10. Pain not of pleuritic or traumatic origin

TREATMENT

- Place patient in a position of comfort (sitting, if no preference).
- O_2 flow rate as indicated by severity of symptoms
- EKG
- IV D_5W TKO
- Treat arrhythmias as indicated.
- Nitroglycerine* only if ordered
- Morphine* only if ordered
- Monitor closely for ST or T wave, or for developing arrhythmias.

See Also:
Arrhythmias

* *See drug section for use*

✱ CONGESTIVE HEART FAILURE

SIGNS AND SYMPTOMS

1. Rales/ronchi
2. Wheezes
3. Dyspnea
4. Cyanosis
5. Coughing up foamy, rust- or blood-colored sputum
6. Tachycardia
7. Unable to sleep supine
8. Paroxysmal nocturnal dyspnea
9. Distended neck veins
10. Exertional dyspnea
11. Patient taking furosemide or digoxin
12. Edema

TREATMENT

- O_2 Max
- Upright position with feet down
- IV D_5W TKO
- Morphine*
- Furosemide (Lasix)*
- Nitroglycerine* (only if morphine is contraindicated)
- Digoxin (Lanoxin)*
- Aminophylline*
- Cardioversion of rapid Atrial-Fibrillation or V-tachy-
- cardia (these arrhythmias may be the cause of pulmonary
- edema)
- PEEP-Intubation
- Rotating tourniquets

* *See drug section for use*

EKG RATE TABLE

SMALL SQUARES R-R	RATE	SMALL SQUARES R-R	RATE
2.5	600	15	(100-)
3	500	16	94
4	375	17½	86
5	(300-)	18	83
6	250	19	79
6½	230	20	(75-)
7	214	21	71
7½	200	22	68
8	188	23	65
8½	176	24	63
9	167	25	(60-)
9½	158	27	56
10	(150-)	28	54
10½	143	30	50-
11	136	35	43-
11½	130	37½	40
12	125	40	38-
12½	120	45	33-
13	115	50	30-
14	107		

Note:

Place positive (LA) lead at the right sternal edge in the 5th intercostal space. Place negative (RA) lead on the upper mid-sternum. Place ground in normal position.

PART TWO
Pulmonary Problems

Airway
Air Embolism
Asthma
Flail Chest
Hemothorax
Pneumothorax
Pulmonary Edema
Pulmonary Embolism
Sucking Chest Wounds
Tension Pneumothorax
Traumatic Asphyxia

FOREIGN BODY (Obstructed)

SIGNS AND SYMPTOMS

1. Little or no air movement
2. Stridor
3. Gagging
4. Cough
5. Hoarseness
6. "Cafe coronary"—inability to speak
7. Cyanosis
8. Coma
9. Respiratory arrest

TREATMENT

- Administer O_2 Max, if partially obstructed (If there is a poor gas exchange, treat as fully obstructed.)
- Abdominal thrusts (times 4)
- Direct visualization
- Perform intubation if foreign body is below vocal cords (attempt to open at least one mainstem).
- Crycothyrotomy†
- ALS and BLS, as indicated

TRACHEAL TRAUMA

SIGNS AND SYMPTOMS

1. Immediate hoarseness
2. Sub-Q air
3. Swollen neck
4. Bruising
5. Decreasing air flow
6. Difficulty swallowing
7. Noisy breathing
8. Coughing up frothy, red blood

TREATMENT

- O_2 Max
- IV, NS
- Intubate (ET-NT) if able
- Monitor vital signs.
- Anticipate respiratory arrest.
- Crycothyrotomy†

† *See same*

continued

CROUP

SIGNS AND SYMPTOMS

1. Age 6 mo. to 3 yr.
2. Cold symptoms for 24 to 48 hrs.
3. Stridor
   - Mild - if "barking" cough heard
   - Moderate - if heard after excitement
   - Severe - if heard at rest
4. Hoarseness
5. Mild respiratory retraction

TREATMENT

- DO NOT attempt to visualize epiglottis.
- Place the patient in position of comfort.
- O_2
- Moist air inhalation
- Racemic epinephrine (Vaponephrine)*

EPIGLOTTITIS

SIGNS AND SYMPTOMS

1. Age 1 to 8 yrs.
2. Sudden onset of cold symptoms (7 to 8 hrs.)
3. Fever
4. Croup type respirations
5. Sore throat
6. Drooling
7. Hoarseness
8. Quiet, anxious, sitting forward

TREATMENT

- DO NOT excite the patient.
- DO NOT attempt to visualize.
- Anticipate obstruction.
- O_2
- Cool, moist air inhalation
- Racemic epinephrine (Vaponephrine)* may be ordered.

** See drug section for use*

continued

- If the patient exhibits a "startle reflex," the airway has obstructed.
  - Administer abdominal thrusts with the patient head down.
  - Mouth-to-mouth resuscitation
  - Intubation
  - Needle or crycothyrotomy† if unable to intubate

CHRONIC OBSTRUCTIVE PULMONARY DISEASE (COPD)

SIGNS AND SYMPTOMS

(Mild)

1. Shortness of breath (SOB)
2. Barrel-chested
3. Costal retraction
4. Distant breath sounds
5. Clubbing fingers
6. Purses

(Moderate)

Any combination of mild and severe distress

(Severe)

All of the above, plus

1. Cough
2. Rales, wheezes, ronchi
3. Cyanosis
4. Signs of cerebral hypoxia
5. Congestive failure

TREATMENT

- O_2 (DO NOT WITHHOLD: BE PREPARED TO VENTILATE PATIENT)
- IV D_5W TKO
- Set the patient upright; lean forward, if tolerated.
- Encourage the patient to cough up secretions.
- Aminophylline*

See Also:

Asthma, hemothorax, congestive failure, pulmonary embolism, tension pneumothorax, flail chest, congestive failure

† *See same*

* *See drug section for use*

SIGNS AND SYMPTOMS

1. Sudden shock
2. Cyanosis
3. Nonpleuritic chest pain
4. SOB
5. Vertigo
6. Open neck or chest injuries
7. Partial paralysis or numbness
8. Seizures
9. Coma
10. Pink, frothy sputum
11. Scuba diving injuries†
12. Improper IV technique

TREATMENT

- Left lateral Trendelenburg position
- O_2 Max (positive pressure)
- IV, NS or LR large bore
- If caused by IV:
  - Clamp off and restart the IV.
  - Keep the IV site at heart level.
- If caused by an open neck wound, apply direct pressure on both ends of vessels involved.
- EKG—Treat arrhythmias as indicated.
- Monitor vital signs and vasopressors, if indicated.

† *See same*

ASTHMA

SIGNS AND SYMPTOMS

1. SOB
2. Wheezing may be absent if the attack is acute and there is little air movement (chest will be hyperinflated).
3. Nonproductive cough (may be productive)
4. Hyperresonant
5. Hyperinflated
6. Accessory muscle use
7. Tachycardia
8. Anxiety

HISTORY

1. Previous attacks
2. Patient medications (to prevent possible patient overdose)
3. Allergies
4. Recent respiratory infection

TREATMENT

- O_2 10 to 15 L/min. with mask and nebulizer
- IV D_5W Max (unless contraindicated)
- Racemic epinephrine (Vaponephrine)*
- Epinephrine*
    - Adult: 0.3 ml to 0.5, 1:1000 sub-Q
    - Ped: 0.1 ml/kg sub-Q
- Aminophylline*
- Monitor EKG for hypoxic or drug-caused changes/dysrhythmias

* *See drug section for use*

FLAIL CHEST

SIGNS AND SYMPTOMS

1. Respiratory distress
2. Multiple rib fractures
3. Paradoxical movement of chest wall (Initially, costal splinting may hide flail section.)
4. Developing pneumothorax/hemothorax
5. Pain with respirations
6. Cyanosis
7. Shock syndrome

TREATMENT

- High flow O_2 (mask)
- IV, NS or LR (large bore)
- Stabilize the flail with 2 to 3 lbs. of sandbags and tape at end of exhalation (use hand to stablize, initially).
- Monitor for associated chest injuries.
- EKG—Monitor for signs of cardiac contusion (BBB/ arrhythmias).

Note:

Due to paradoxical movement of the chest wall, air is shunted between the affected and unaffected sides. Despite Kussmaul respiration, little air is moved externally. Distress develops rapidly. Fractures of first-second-third ribs usually are fatal due to associated injury. Seventy-five percent of fatal accident victims have chest injuries.

HEMOTHORAX

SIGNS AND SYMPTOMS

1. Penetrating or blunt chest trauma
2. Fractured ribs
3. SOB
4. Decreased breath sounds on affected side
5. Distended neck veins
6. Cyanosis
7. Shock syndrome
8. Dull percussion on affected side
9. Complication of tension pneumothorax decompression
10. Spontaneous pneumothorax

TREATMENT

- O_2 Max
- IV, NS or LR (2 or more, if needed)
- Apply MAST only with physician's orders.
- Decompress as for tension pneumothorax. †
- Monitor for decreased vitals and associated chest injuries.
- Treat rib fractures or flails.

† *See same*

SIGNS AND SYMPTOMS

1. SOB
2. Chest pain
3. Decreased breath sounds on affected side
4. Cyanosis
5. Shock syndrome
6. History of:
   - Sudden onset after coughing, exercise or rapid altitude change
   - Previous respiratory problems (TB, emphysema, COPD)
   - Fractured ribs
   - Blunt chest trauma
7. Tracheal shift toward affected side

TREATMENT

- High flow O_2
- Splint fractured ribs.
- IV, NS or LR large bore, TKO (unless signs of shock)
- Monitor closely for worsening of symptoms.

See Also:

Hemothorax, tension pneumothorax, flail chest, cardiac contusion

PULMONARY EDEMA

SIGNS AND SYMPTOMS

1. Dyspnea
2. Rales/ronchi
3. Cyanosis
4. Tachycardia
5. Frothy sputum (may be blood-tinged)
6. Shock syndrome
7. Distended neck veins
8. Arrhythmia
9. Hypotension

HISTORY

1. Vigorous activity at altitude in unacclimatized persons
2. Inhalation of noxious or hot gases
3. Near-drowning
4. Cardiac arrhythmias or failure
5. Aspiration
6. Blunt chest trauma
7. Overhydration
8. Sepsis
9. Narcotic overdose
10. Heatstroke
11. Fever
12. Neurogenic causes
13. Renal disease
14. AMI
15. Anemia

TREATMENT

- O_2 Max
- Place patient with feet down, unless contraindicated.
- IV D_5W TKO
- Morphine* (unless narcotic overdose is cause)
- Furosemide (Lasix)*
- Aminophylline*
- Intubation and PEEP
- EKG
- Rotating tourniquets (contraindicated if anemia is present)

* *See drug section for use*

continued

SIGNS AND SYMPTOMS

Sudden onset of:

1. Anxiety
2. Dyspnea
3. Tachycardia
4. Tachypnea
5. Cyanosis
6. Shock syndrome
7. Distended neck veins
8. Pulmonary edema
9. Hemoptysis
10. Rales/wheezes
11. Pleuritic chest pain
12. Hypoxic seizures
13. Coma/death

HISTORY

1. Sudden onset of signs and symptoms
2. Recent surgery
3. Pregnancy/postpartum
4. Oral contraceptive use
5. Phlebitis
6. Fractures (usually long bone)
7. Varicose veins
8. Congestive failure
9. Arrhythmias (i.e.—atrial fibrillation)
10. Prolonged bed rest
11. Acute infections
12. Obesity
13. Prosthetic heart valves

TREATMENT

- O_2 Max and suction to aid in maintaining a patent airway
- IV, TKO
- EKG—Treat arrhythmias.
- Vasopressor
- Administer an analgesic in absence of shock.
- Elevate the patient's legs.

Note:

Seventy-five percent of embolism originates from veins in the lower extremities.

OPEN PNEUMOTHORAX

SIGNS AND SYMPTOMS

1. Chest wound with air moving in and out with respiration
2. Acute respiratory distress signs
3. Sucking or slurping sounds
4. Marked cyanosis

If the wound is larger than the size of the glottis, ALL air enters the chest there (rapidly fatal, as no air enters alveoli).

TREATMENT

- Quickly seal the sucking wound on forced expiration with the patient's mouth and nose closed (use hand until dressing can be applied). Use several layers of petroleum gauze or cellophane on 3½ sides only.
- O_2 Max
- IV, NS
- Monitor for decreasing vital signs and tension pneumothorax. †
- Loosen the dressing if tension develops.
- Splint fractured ribs.

† *See same*

TENSION PNEUMOTHORAX *

SIGNS AND SYMPTOMS

1. Blunt or penetrating injury (rarely spontaneous)
2. SOB
3. Decreased breath sounds on affected side
4. Sub-Q air
5. Distended neck veins
6. Tracheal shift away from injured side
7. Costal bulging
8. Cyanosis
9. Shock
10. Tachypnea
11. Drumlike percussion on affected side
12. The intubated patient shows signs of increasing resistance to the mask with an unobstructed tube and without a distended abdomen.

TREATMENT

- O_2 Max
- IV
- Decompress
  - Expose and clean anterior axillary or midclavicular #5 rib (nipple line).
  - Hit the rib with a needle; then slide the needle over the rib.
  - Remove the needle and attach a Heimlich valve or an IV tubing, and partly empty the IV bag placed below the level of the patient.
  - This procedure is very painful; expect resistance from the patient (restrain if necessary).
- Splint fractured ribs.

Note:

If tension develops after sealing a sucking chest wound, loosen the dressing.

See Also:

Pneumothorax, hemothorax

TRAUMATIC ASPHYXIA

SIGNS AND SYMPTOMS

1. Crushing type injury to chest (usually with sternal fracture or flail chest)
2. Marked cyanosis of head, face and neck with definite demarcation
3. Petechiae
4. Swollen tongue/lips
5. Bulging or protruding, blood-shot eyes
6. Distended neck veins
7. Severe shock
8. Signs of cerebral edema
9. Coma

TREATMENT

- High flow O_2
- Multiple large IV's
- MAST
- Monitor for chest injuries.
- Dexamethasone (Decadron)*

* *See drug section for use*

PART THREE
Environmental Emergencies

Anaphylactic Reaction
Alcohol Abuse
Burns
Cold Exposure
Diving Injuries
Drowning/Near Drowning
Eye Injuries
Fractures
Head Injuries
Heat Exposure

STAGES OF DELIRIUM TREMENS (D.T.'s)

1. Shakes, increased pulse and Bp, blurred vision
2. Hallucinations
3. Agitation, amnesia, disorientation, delusions
4. Seizures, coma, death

Alcoholics may have one or more of the following associated problems:

1. Antabuse—alcohol reactions
2. Toxic alcohol O.D.
3. Pneumonia
4. Hepatic dysfunctions
5. Ulcers
6. Esophageal ruptures
7. Hypoglycemia
8. Seizures
9. Falling injuries
10. Aspiration
11. Acute myocardial infarction (AMI)
12. Decreased pain reactions

TREATMENT

- ABC's
- IV
- O_2
- $D_{50}W$*
- As indicated, by exam, for secondary problems
- Valium to control seizures

ANTABUSE (Disulfiram)—ALCOHOL REACTIONS

SIGNS AND SYMPTOMS

1. Flushed skin
2. Headache
3. Dypsnea
4. Nausea and vomiting
5. Salivation

Progresses to:

6. Profound shock
7. Cyanosis
8. Coma

(Symptoms usually start one-half hr. after ingestion.)

* *See drug section for use*

continued

TREATMENT (Severe)

- O_2
- IV, NS or LR
- MAST, if indicated
- Diphenhydramine (Benadryl)*
- Monitor for EKG changes
- Diazepam (Valium)*

TREATMENT (Mild)

- O_2
- Oral antihistamines

TOXIC ALCOHOL O.D. (Methyl, Wood)

SIGNS AND SYMPTOMS

1. Headache
2. Nausea and vomiting
3. Gastric pain
4. Dilated, sluggish pupils
5. Visual disturbances/blindness
6. Shortness of breath (SOB)
7. Cyanosis

Severe cases exhibit a greater degree of the above, plus:

8. Hyperexcitability
9. Seizures
10. Hypotension

TREATMENT

- ABC's
- IV, NS or LR
- O_2
- Sodium Bicarbonate*
- Ethyl alcohol (whiskey) 30 ml q 3 to 4 hrs.

* *See drug section for use*

✱ ANAPHYLACTIC REACTION

SIGNS AND SYMPTOMS

1. Anxiety
2. Dyspnea
3. Wheezing, sneezing, stridor, hoarseness
4. Facial edema
5. Pounding headache
6. Itching
7. Hives
8. Abdominal cramps
9. Tachycardia
10. Bright red skin (rash may not be seen due to edema)
11. Hx of recent:
    - Medications
    - Bee sting
    - Allergic exposures
12. Profound shock
13. Seizures

TREATMENT (Mild)

- Sub-Q Epinephrine* 0.3, 1:1000
- O_2 high flow, 10 to 15 L/min.
- IV
- Diphenhydramine (Benadryl)*

TREATMENT (Severe)

- O_2
- IV, NS or D_5W
- 10 cc 1:10,000 EPI IV
- Without IV: EPI sublingual or transtracheally
- Diphenhydramine (Benadryl)*

* *See drug section for use*

continued

BEE STING

TREATMENT (Severe)

- ABC's (intubation oral-nasal)
- Remove the stinger.
- Apply a tourniquet above the site, if possible.
- O_2
- 0.5cc 1:1000 sub-Q below tourniquet and 0.5cc, 1:1000 sub-Q in arm on opposite side of body (NEVER inject EPI into a finger or toe)
- IV, NS or LR
- Diphenhydramine (Benadryl)*
- Aminophylline*
- If hypotension persists: Dopamine or Metaraminol*

** See drug section for use*

BURNS

HISTORY

1. Type of burn
2. Extent of burn
3. Steam vs. open flame
4. Closed space vs. open space (high concentration of CO_2, toxic gases and smoke)
5. Respiratory involvement
   - Singed nasal hair
   - Facial burns
   - Sputum or soot in nose
   - Cough
   - Wheeze/ronchi
   - Hoarseness
   - Dyspnea
6. Associated trauma or illnesses
7. Prior causes (i.e.—AMI, O.D., seizure, diabetes, coma)

THERMAL

TREATMENT

- Stop burning process. Remove affected clothes, cutting around adherent areas. Wash entire burned area with sterile water or saline. DO NOT ALLOW THE PATIENT TO CHILL.
- Establish an airway; ET-NT, if indicated. Monitor for upper airway edema.
- IV, NS or LR
- Remove rings or other constricting items. Check distal circulation.
- Apply a dry dressing if the burned area is large (moist for smaller areas).
- O_2 4 to 6 L/min. nasal, unless respiratory involvement is present, then Max
- Administer an analgesic, if ordered.
- Monitor for edema affecting distal circulation, EKG and signs of respiratory involvement.

CHEMICAL

TREATMENT

- Brush off dry chemicals.
- Wash with copious amounts of water.
- Apply a moist dressing.

continued

- Monitor for edema affecting distal circulation and signs of intoxication from chemical absorption.
- O_2
- IV, as per thermal burn
- Administer an analgesic, if ordered.

ELECTRICAL

TREATMENT

- Protect yourself and other rescuers.
- Remove the patient from the electrical source.
- ALS as indicated by EKG
- Locate entrance and exit wounds.
- Apply necessary dressings.
- Monitor for edema affecting distal circulation.
- Administer an analgesic, if ordered.
- Monitor for EKG changes/arrhythmias. Administer prophylactic lidocaine*, if indicated/ordered.

Note:

A. Peds and elderly shock fast

B. Splint hand in burn position with thumb parallel to fingers

C. Suspect AMI or toxic gases in burned firefighter

** See drug section for use*

CLASSIFICATION OF BURNS

MINOR:
First degree burns over less than 20% of body area; second degree burns over less than 15%; third degree burns over less than 2%.

MODERATE:
First degree burns over more than 20% of body area; second degree burns over more than 15%; third degree burns over more than 2%.

SEVERE:
Second degree burns over more than 30% of body area; third degree burns over more than 10%; OR burns associated with fracture, respiratory tract, genitalia, hands, feet or secondary causes.

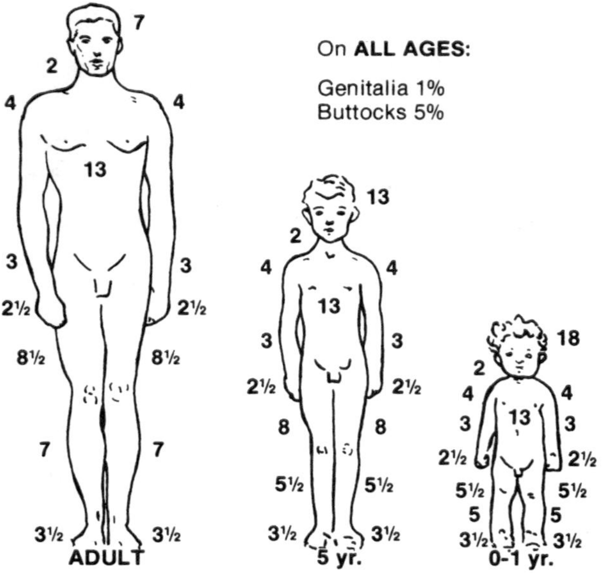

On **ALL AGES:**

Genitalia 1%
Buttocks 5%

Note:
The percentage of body surface for the posterior torso is the same as that indicated for the anterior torso.

HYPOTHERMIA

PROGRESSION OF STAGES:

1. Apathy
2. Uncoordination
3. Uncontrolled shivering
4. Sleepiness
5. Shivering stops
6. Coma
7. Pulse and respiration decreases

TREATMENT

- Remove wet clothing.
- If unconscious:
  - Apply hot packs to kidneys, groin and neck
  - Heated O_2
  - Thermal blanket
  - Warm gastric lavage
- For conscious patients, ambulate, if at all able, and give hot fluids.
- EKG
- O_2
- IV D_5W TKO
- Watch the patient carefully if body temperature is below 87°F (liable to V-fibrillate as temperature rises past 87°).
- Treat any frostbite.

FROSTBITE

SIGNS AND SYMPTOMS

1. Red and inflamed
2. Gray or mottled
3. Frozen and white
4. Pain progressing to parathesia

TREATMENT

- Immerse in 106° to 110° F water.
- DO NOT massage.
- NO SMOKING OR ALCOHOL
- DO NOT allow to refreeze.

DECOMPRESSION DISEASE

"The Bends" are caused by too rapid of an ascent from deep water; however, they can occur in less than 33 feet of water or during a rapid altitude change in an inadequately pressurized aircraft.

SIGNS AND SYMPTOMS

1. Joint pain
2. SOB
3. Dizziness
4. Fatigue
5. Speech and/or visual disturbances
6. Paralysis/numbness
7. Headache
8. Seizures
9. Coma

(Most divers have onset of symptoms within 30 min. to 6 hrs., occasionally 24 to 48 hrs.)

Note:

A. Any diver with complaint of symptoms and a history of diving injuries within 48 hrs. should be treated for decompression disease.

B. All seriously injured divers who were not decompressed on ascent due to extent of injury should be treated for decompression disease.

TREATMENT

- Recompression
- High flow O_2
- IV
- Left lateral Trendelenburg position

continued

"THE SQUEEZE"

SIGNS AND SYMPTOMS

1. Breath holding on descent causes sudden sharp local pain in:
   - GI tract
   - Chest
   - Ears
   - Sinuses
   - Teeth
2. Edema
3. Bleeding
4. Rupture of hollow internal organs

TREATMENT

- Treat the patient for indicated injury, including ruptured bowel, pneumothorax and tension pneumothorax.

GAS INTOXICATION — Carbon monoxide

SIGNS AND SYMPTOMS

1. Dizziness
2. Euphoria
3. Pink-red lips and mouth

TREATMENT

- ABC's, CPR
- High flow O_2
- Administer hyperbaric O_2 at 3 atmospheres for 1 hr.

GAS INTOXICATION — Carbon dioxide

SIGNS AND SYMPTOMS

1. Dizziness
2. Lethargy
3. SOB
4. Coma

TREATMENT

- ABC's, CPR
- High flow O_2

DROWNING/NEAR DROWNING

SOME CAUSES:

1. Nonswimmer
2. Alcohol/drugs
3. Diving injuries
4. Hyperventilation
5. Seizures
6. Hypothermia
7. Suicide
8. Exhaustion
9. Diving reflex

TREATMENT

- Airway/O_2 (frequent suctioning required)
- CPR/ALS as indicated
- Suspect head/neck injury.
- NG tube
- PEEP
- Suspect/treat possible causes of drowning ($D_{50}W$*, naloxone*).

(All near drownings, even those without secondary complications, should be transported to a hospital due to possible delayed onset of pulmonary edema or respiratory infections.)

** See drug section for use*

PENETRATING OR RUPTURING

TREATMENT

- Avoid contaminating the eye (use sterile gloves).
- Immobilize the object if still impaled; do not use pressure.
- Put nothing directly on the surface of the injured eye.
- Use an eye cup or eye guard.
- Cover both eyes.
- Cause no increased intraoccular pressure.
- Transport sitting in the absence of retinal detachment or other contraindications.
- NPO
- Check past visual history.

NONPENETRATING

These injuries may result from foreign bodies, welding burns, sun burns, corneal abrasions, or contact lens irritation.

TREATMENT

- Remove the object with a moist, cotton-tipped applicator.
- Bandage both eyes with slight pressure.

THERMAL BURNS

TREATMENT

- Wash the eyes gently.
- Cover both eyes with moist dressings.

CHEMICAL BURNS

TREATMENT

- Continuous irrigation

CENTRAL RETINAL ARTERY OCCLUSION

This condition involves sudden, painless visual loss to one eye that is usually nontraumatic. The patient has only light perception in the affected eye. The pupil is nonreactive, but it will respond ALONG WITH the unaffected pupil.

TREATMENT

- Put pressure over the eyeball with the heel of a hand for one hour (may cause a vagal reaction; monitor for EKG changes).

continued

RETINAL DETACHMENT

This injury involves traumatic injury to the eye or head that causes the patient to see only light flashes or a curtain-blocking vision. The patient may see dark spots.

TREATMENT

- Patch both eyes.
- Gently transport the patient SUPINE.

HYPHEMA

This injury involves a history of direct trauma to the eye (fist, BB or baseball). The patient sees red. There is a red fluid level visible across the iris.

TREATMENT

- Patch both eyes.
- Apply an ice pack.

SIGNS AND SYMPTOMS

1. Pain
2. Swelling
3. Ecchymosis
4. Deformity/angulation
5. Crepitus (Do not elicit this sign!)
6. Guarding and splinting
7. Open wounds
8. Protruding bone ends
9. Associated injuries
10. Distal embarrassment

TREATMENT (Open)

- Control bleeding.
  - Dress the wound before splinting.
  - Use a tourniquet as a last resort for traumatic amputation or a limb mangled beyond salvage.
- •• Straighten severely angulated fractures, UNLESS A JOINT IS INVOLVED: perform a field reduction only if there is no distal circulation.
- •• Use a padded splint and immobilize the joint above and below.
- •• Monitor the patient for associated injury.
- •• Check distal circulation or neurological changes due to swelling inside splint.
- •• Apply ice and elevate the fracture.
- •• An IV may be required for a femur fracture or for shock.

TREATMENT (Closed)

- See • • steps under FRACTURE TREATMENT (Open).

TREATMENT (Dislocations)

- See • • steps under FRACTURE TREATMENT (Open).
- Field reduction should be performed ONLY if transport time is greater than 2 hrs. and there is no distal pulse.

Note:

A. Always splint a hand in position of function (slight flexion, fingers spread slightly and thumb able to meet index finger tip; leave finger tips exposed).

B. Children have a high incidence of ruptured spleen associated with femur fracture.

HEAD INJURIES

SIGNS AND SYMPTOMS

1. Mechanism of injury—recent blow to head
2. Lucid interval
3. Headache
4. Nausea/vomiting
5. Disorientation
6. Decreasing level of consciousness
7. Signs of skull fracture
   - Deformity
   - Hematoma
   - Contusions/lacerations
   - Blood/CSF from ears/nose
   - Racoon eyes/battle sign
   - Localized pain
8. Neurological defects
9. Pathologic, abnormal, asymmetrical reflexes
10. Pupil changes unassociated with eye related problems/ medications
11. Eyes wander/deviate from midline
12. Respiratory patterning
13. Posturing/seizures
14. Temperature changes
15. Increasing Bp, falling pulse
16. Coma

TREATMENT

- Protect the patient's neck.
- Insure a continued, adequate airway.
- Hyperventilate with O_2
- Place in side position with head of board elevated.
- IV—large bore TKO (Pure head injury seldom is the cause of profound shock.)
- Draw required blood for lab work.
- Check and record neuro status frequently.
- Expect vomiting.
- No nasal suction, if CSF present
- Dexamethasone (Decadron)*
- Furosemide (Lasix)*
- Mannitol 25% *

* *See drug section for use*

HEAT STROKE

SIGNS AND SYMPTOMS

1. Headache/dizziness
2. Nausea
3. Hot/dry skin
4. Temperature of 105° F+
5. Thirst/dryness of the mouth
6. Bounding pulse—progressing to weak, thin pulse
7. Arrhythmias
8. Syncope/seizures
9. Coma/death

Predisposing factors include: elderly, hemiplegia, obesity, infirmity, diuretics, sedatives, atropine, alcoholism, previous febrile illness

TREATMENT

- Airway and O_2
- Cool the patient rapidly to a rectal temperature of 102° F, then remove to cool environment.
- EKG
- IV D_5W TKO
- Diazepam (Valium)* to control seizures
- Monitor for secondary complications (CHF, AMI, CVA, DIC, pulmonary edema, arrhythmias, kidney dysfunction).

* *See drug section for use*

continued

CRAMPS (usually due to salt depletion)

SIGNS AND SYMPTOMS

1. Normal temperature
2. Excessive diaphoresis
3. Severe muscle pains or spasms

TREATMENT

- Remove the patient to a cool environment.
- IV, NS or 1 teaspoon of salt in a glass of juice, if available.
- DO NOT give the patient plain water.
- AVOID SALT TABLETS.

EXHAUSTION (salt depletion plus dehydration)

SIGNS AND SYMPTOMS

1. Temperature normal or low
2. Excess diaphoresis
3. Pale, clammy skin
4. Syncope/dizziness
5. Nausea and vomiting

TREATMENT

- Treat as for cramps, but give nothing by mouth.

PART FOUR
Medical Emergencies

ACUTE ABDOMEN

SIGNS AND SYMPTOMS

1. Pain
   - type
   - location
   - radiating/referred
   - onset
   - aggravating/alleviating
2. Guarding
3. Distension
4. Nausea/vomiting
5. Bloody stools or vomitus
6. Tachycardia
7. Orthostatic hypotension/decreasing Bp
8. Penetrating wounds
9. History of blunt trauma
10. Abdominal/kidney bruises
11. Polyuria, hemouria, dysuria
12. Pregnancy or abnormal mensus
13. Diarrhea
14. Pallor
15. Shock syndrome

TREATMENT

- IV, NS LR large bore (2 or more if needed)
- Apply MAST and inflate, if needed.
- O_2
- Place the patient in a side position, if tolerated.
- EXPECT VOMITING.
- NG tube may be ordered.

Note:

Protruding intestines should be washed with NS and a sterile dressing should be applied. If transport time is greater than 15 minutes, wash the intestines with NS, re-insert and cover with a dressing.

THORACIC

SIGNS AND SYMPTOMS

1. Chest pain; excruciating or tearing in nature
2. Orthopnea
3. Shock syndrome
4. Unilateral absence of major pulses
5. Unequal blood pressure in arms
6. Pulsation at sternoclavicular joint
7. Murmur
8. Possible history of hypertension or arteriosclerotic heart disease

TREATMENT

- Place the patient upright and slightly reclining.
- O_2
- IV, multiple large bore TKO, unless shock is profound
- Uninflated MAST (inflate if the patient is comatose)

ABDOMINAL

SIGNS AND SYMPTOMS

1. Pain, excruciating or tearing, radiating to back
2. Shock syndrome
3. Pulsating, expansile abdominal mass
4. Embarrassed circulation to one or both legs

TREATMENT

- O_2
- IV, multiple large bore TKO, unless shock is profound
- Uninflated MAST (inflate if the patient is comatose)

CEREBROVASCULAR ACCIDENT (CVA)

PREDISPOSING CAUSES

40 years or older, female on birth control pills, negro youth with sickle cell disease, heart disease, arrhythmias, atherosclerosis, hypertension, infection, fractures, thrombosis (see also embolism) and diabetes

SIGNS AND SYMPTOMS

1. History includes predisposing causes or transient ischemic attack (T.I.A.)
2. Headache
3. Hypertension
4. Focal neurologic findings (usually one-sided)
   - Numbness/paralysis
   - Facial droop
   - Unequal reflexes
   - Pathological reflexes
   - Unequal pupils
   - One-sided seizures
5. Confusion/agitation
6. Facial flush
7. Speech, visual, hearing or smell changes
8. Bruit (may be intermittent)
9. Nuchal rigidity
10. Coma (usually has a cause other than stroke)
11. Respiratory patterning
12. Temperature changes

TREATMENT

- Insure a continued adequate airway and administer O_2.
- EKG
- IV D_5W TKO ‡
- Draw blood for lab analysis.
- Elevate the patient's head.

‡ Treat shock, if present.
- Fluid challenge
- MAST
- Vasopressors

INSULIN SHOCK

SIGNS AND SYMPTOMS

1. Headache
2. Hunger
3. Irrational or confused behavior
4. Uncoordination
5. Weakness
6. Visual disturbances, usually diplopia
7. Shock syndrome (Bp usually normal; pulse rapid or normal)
8. Hx
   - On insulin
   - Nothing eaten
   - Excess stress, exercise or alcohol
9. Seizures
10. Coma

TREATMENT

- Airway—O_2
- Dextrostix®
- Draw and hold blood.
- IV D_5W
- $D_{50}W$*
- EKG

* *See drug section for use*

continued

KETOACIDOSIS

SIGNS AND SYMPTOMS

1. Fever
2. Thirst
3. Polyurea
4. Dehydration
5. Hot, dry skin
6. Kussmaul respirations
7. Acetone odor
8. Nausea and vomiting
9. Abdominal cramps
10. Elevated glucose on Dextrostix®
11. Coma (late)
12. Shock syndrome due to dehydration (late)

TREATMENT

- If in doubt due to similarity of late symptoms, treat as for insulin shock.
- IV, NS
- EKG (for potassium level changes)
- O_2

1. Physical exam
2. Level of consciousness—
   GLASGOW COMA SCALE (one score per group)

MOTOR

Points

6	Obeys simple commands
5	Localizes noxious stimulus
4	Reacts to noxious stimulus
3	Decordicate to stimulus
2	Decerebrate to stimulus
1	No motor response (in absence of spinal injury)

VERBAL

Points

5	Conscious-alert-oriented (CAO) to person, place and time
4	Confused
3	Nonconversive; reacts with confused or one-word verbal response
2	Nonintelligent words or sounds
1	No verbal response

EYE MOVEMENT

Points

4	Open spontaneously
3	Open to verbal stimulus
2	Open to noxious stimulus
1	No response

Note:

(A total score of 7 or less qualifies as COMA.)

3. Loss of consciousness (Was there a lucid interval?)
4. Sensation and motion in all extremities
   - Reflexes
   - Pathologic reflexes (i.e.—Clonus, Babinski . . .)
5. Respiratory rate and pattern
6. Pupil reaction and eye movements

continued

7. Facial nerve test (if conscious)
- Follows fingers with eyes only
- Closes eyes tightly
- Big smile; big frown
- Bites jaws together (Palpate masseter muscles; note if they are unequal.)
- Sticks tongue out and moves it from side to side

8. History

Include:
- Headache
- Nausea and vomiting
- Dizziness
- Visual disturbances

REPORT

Type/name of agent
Route of exposure:
- Ingestion
- Inhalation
- Absorbed
- Injection

Amount/duration of exposure
Time of exposure
Other medications/alcohol
Reason for/cause of
Level of consciousness
Symptoms: ______________________________

____

Physical exam and medical history

TREATMENT

- Protect EMS personnel from hazards.
- Insure continued adequate respirations; administer O_2.
- Contact MD or Poison Control
- Remove contaminant
  - Remove to safe atmosphere
  - Flush skin/hair 20 minutes
  - Empty stomach (Ipecac†)
  - If poison was injected, venous tourniquet above site
- IV, large bore (Draw required blood for lab work.)
  Hypotensive:
  - Fluid challenge
  - MAST
  - Vasopressor
- Unconscious
  - $D_{50}W$*
  - Naloxone (Narcan)*

† *See same*
* *See drug section for use*

✱ SEIZURES

ETIOLOGY

CVA, hypoxia, hypoglycemia, fever, head injury, idiopathic, congenital, meningitis, poisons, overdoses, withdrawal

TYPES

1. Status Epilepticus - seizure longer than 5 min. or two isolated seizures without lucid interval (requires urgent treatment)
2. Jacksonian - starts one place and spreads
3. Focal Motor - one body part
4. Psychomotor - altered personality
5. Grand Mal - general body involvement
6. Petit Mal - LOC (loss of consciousness) without motor loss
7. Febrile - associated with fever (usually neonatal or pediatric
8. Hysterical - audience present, no injury or incontinence
9. Neonatal - may present as facial twitching, apneic episodes, rigidity, chewing, blinking, flexion/extension of trunk (Neonatal seizures have a high mortality rate.)

HISTORY

1. Previous seizures
2. Medication
3. When did the last seizure occur?
4. Describe start of seizure and type of activity
5. Did the patient have syncope first?
6. Recent injury, O.D., alcohol use or irregular rhythm

continued

COMPLICATIONS

1. Aspiration
2. Fractures
3. Oral trauma
4. Bruises, hematomas
5. Sprains
6. Altered states
7. Hallucinations
8. Agitation

TREATMENT

- Protect the patient from self-injury.
- Administer O_2.
- Establish an IV.
- Blood to hold/Dextrostix®
- Diazepam (Valium), phenytoin or phenobarbital*
- EKG—Treat arrhythmias.
- $D_{50}W$ *
- Control fever (tepid bath only—NO ALCOHOL BATHS).
- Treat associated injuries.

* *See drug section for use*

SEPSIS

ETIOLOGY

Prolonged infection, meningitis, pneumonia, dental abscesses, UTI, use of dirty needle by drug abusers, IV contaminations and blood transfusion

SIGNS AND SYMPTOMS (Early)

1. Chills
2. Fever
3. Warm, dry, flushed skin
4. Slight tachycardia
5. Normal or mild hypotension
6. Lethargy (occasionally alert)

SIGNS AND SYMPTOMS (Late)

1. Subnormal temperature
2. Shock syndrome

TREATMENT

- O_2—Establish airway.
- IV, NS (In late shock, a fluid challenge may be ordered)
- Sodium bicarbonate*
- EKG
- Dopamine (Intropin)* is pressor of choice
- Monitor for pulmonary edema and/or distending neck veins.

* *See drug section for use*

TYPES

1. Hypovolemic—Decreased fluid due to internal or external blood loss, or to dehydration from: nausea and vomiting, burns, fever or ketoacidosis
2. Capacitance—Increased vessel space due to: spinal/neuro causes, toxins (sepsis), O.D. or fainting
3. Cardiogenic—Pump failure from AMI
4. Insulin—Hypoglycemia
5. Obstructive—Mechanical restriction to flow from: tension pneumothorax, tamponade, or supine hypotension syndrome in pregnancy

SIGNS AND SYMPTOMS

1. Anxiety/dizziness
2. Decreasing blood pressure/orthostatic hypotension
3. Increasing pulse (may not be rapid in certain cardiac conditions, patients taking certain medications or in late stages of shock)
4. Tachypnea
5. Pallor
6. Cyanosis
7. Skin temperature (Warm)
   - Sepsis
   - Arsenic poisoning
   - Spinal/neurological damage
   - Vasodilator drugs

   Skin temperature (Cool)
   - Blood loss
   - Insulin shock
   - Late sepsis
   - Anaphylaxis
8. Diaphoresis
9. Dull, lusterless, dilated pupils
10. Nausea and vomiting
11. Lethargy/decreasing mental status
12. Poor capillary refilling
13. Rash/hives (Anaphylaxsis†)
14. Wounds or infections (Sepsis†)

† *See same*

continued

TREATMENT

- Insure continued adequate airway.
- O_2 Max (Assist shallow respirations.)
- Multiple large bore IV's, NS or LR—titrate to need
- Apply MAST.
- Treat underlying causes.
- Keep the patient warm (not hot).
- 50meq sodium bicarbonate* for every 2000cc's of fluid given may be ordered.
- $D_{50}W$*
- Narcan*
- EKG

* *See drug section for use*

TREATMENT

- ABC's
- Splint the patient's neck.
- O_2
- Monitor vital signs and EKG.
- Large bore IV D_5W TKO
- Draw and hold blood.
- Dextrostix®
  - Greater than 45mg%, go to next step
  - Less than 45mg%, give $D_{50}W$*
    - Adult: 50cc
    - Ped: 1cc/kg
- Narcan*
  - Adult: 0.4mg
  - Ped: 0.01mg/kg
- Treat for hypovolemia; MAST; multiple IV's

NOMAGRAM: For causes of COMA

A—Accidents, acidosis, airway, alcohol
E—Electrocution, embolism, epilepsy, electrolytes
I—Ingestion, intoxication, inhalation
O—O.D.
U—Uremia
H—Head, heart, hypoxia, hypovolemia
I—Insulin, infection
T—Thermal, trauma
S—Stroke, sepsis

* *See drug section for use*

PART FIVE
Pediatrics and OB/GYN Problems

APGAR SCORE

	0	1	2
Appearance (color)	blue/pale	cyanotic extremities only	pink
Pulse	0	Below 100	Over 100
Grimace mild noxious reacts to stimulus	0	facial grimace	crys
Activity	limp	weak	active
Respiratory	0	less than 25	25 to 40*

Score the patient at 0 and 5 minutes.

A score less than 6 means that the patient is in distress and should be monitored closely.

A respiratory rate greater than 60 indicates that the patient is experiencing respiratory distress.

Transport vs. Field Delivery

1. Previous child births (first is usually slower)
2. Contraction Frequency
   - Longer than 5 minutes usually allows time to transport
   - Less than 2 minutes (not first child) means impending delivery
3. Has the amnionic sac ruptured? **When?** (Risk of infection increases with time between rupture and delivery. Advise the physician of this.)
4. Does the mother need to move her bowels? Advise her that this is normal (delivery is eminent).
5. Is crowning present? If so, control the rate of delivery and proceed as per indications (i.e.—breech, prolapsed cord, etc.).

NORMAL:

Large bore IV, if time allows
DO NOT allow the mother to go to the bathroom.
DO NOT restrain or delay delivery.

- Drape
- Tell the mother to pant during contractions.
- Control the rate of delivery.
- Check the amnionic sac for rupture.
- Suction the baby's nose and mouth before shoulder delivery, if possible (especially if meconium is present in the amnionic fluid—meconium aspiration †).
- If the umbilical cord is around the baby's neck, tie it twice and cut between the ties.
- Apply downward traction to aid in delivering the upper shoulder.
- Apply upward traction to aid in delivering the lower shoulder.
- Place the baby's head lower than the body.
- Suction frequently.
- Record the Apgar score and note the time of birth.
- Place the baby on the mother's abdomen, head down.
- After the cord has stopped pulsating, cut and tie the cord 8 inches from the naval.
- Deliver and retain the placenta. Never pull on the umbilical cord to deliver the placenta.
- Massage the uterus to slow bleeding.
- Place a pad over the vagina.

† *See same*

MULTIPLE BIRTHS

TREATMENT

- Assemble extra equipment and hands.
- Proceed with the delivery as indicated.
- When the first child delivers, tie and cut the umbilical cord (prevents hemorrhage of the twin).
- If the second baby has not delivered in 10 minutes, transport the mother to the hospital.
- Multiple birth babies tend to be small and should be treated as if premature.

PREMATURE

TREATMENT

- Expect the baby to be in distress.
- Suction frequently and well, but do not compromise oxygenation; stop if the baby's pulse begins to slow.
- KEEP THE BABY WARM AND DRY.
- Check the umbilical cord frequently for bleeding; place a second tie if indicated.
- O_2 by tent
- Keep the baby's environment as sterile as possible to avoid infections.

MECONIUM ASPIRATION

TREATMENT

- Be prepared to suction the infant using a DeLee trap as soon as the head is delivered, but before the body presents.
- If the baby's airway has not been suctioned before the onset of respirations:
  - Intubate the baby.
  - Using the ET tube, apply suction directly as you remove the tube.
  - Repeat as above.
  - If meconium is exceptionally thick, 1 to 2ml of NS should be instilled in the ET tube before suctioning.

Note:

Any delivery in which the amnionic fluid is stained with meconium should be treated as if aspiration has occurred.

continued

BREECH

TREATMENT

- Procedures are the same as for normal delivery, but expect the baby to need CPR/ALS.
- Support the trunk and buttocks, and control the rate of head delivery.
- If the baby's head takes longer than 3 minutes to deliver, make an airway using two fingers of a gloved hand inserted into the vagina, and try to relieve pressure on the umbilical cord.
- Proceed as above.
- If there are no results within 3 minutes, maintain the airway and transport immediately.
- If one foot or arm delivers, transport immediately. DO NOT PULL the baby out.
- Place the mother in the knee chest position or in the high shock position on the left side.

PROLAPSED CORD

TREATMENT

- Place the mother in knee/chest position or supine with a pillow elevating her hips.
- Place a gloved hand into the vagina with the other hand on the abdomen and push the baby's head up about 3 inches. Remain in this position until the baby has been surgically delivered.
- Do not replace the cord (cover with a sterile, moist dressing).
- O_2 high concentration (mother)
- DO NOT push the cord back into the vagina.
- Check the cord for pulses.

EXCESSIVE POSTPARTUM BLEEDING

TREATMENT

- Multiple large IV's with blood y's
- Massage the uterus.
- MAST
- O_2
- Oxytocin (Pitocin)*

** See drug section for use*

continued

PROLAPSED UTERUS (Uterine Inversion)

TREATMENT

- Place the patient supine.
- O_2
- Multiple large bore IV's NS/LR—Draw blood for type and cross.
- MAST if shock is profound
- DO NOT remove the attached placenta
- Make one attempt to replace the uterus manually by exerting pressure on the area closest to the cervix.
- If unable to replace the uterus, treat the patient as for an eviserated bowel.

THREATENED ABORTION

SIGNS AND SYMPTOMS

1. Bleeding in early pregnancy
2. Pain (comparable to menstrual cramps)

INEVITABLE ABORTION

SIGNS AND SYMPTOMS

1. Bleeding (may be massive)
2. Symptoms of pregnancy may have disappeared.
3. Uterine contractions

INCOMPLETE ABORTION

SIGNS AND SYMPTOMS

1. Passing of part of the products of conception
2. Bleeding
3. Symptoms of pregnancy may have disappeared.

TREATMENT FOR ABORTION

- O_2
- IV, NS large bore (multiple if indicated)
- MAST if shock is profound
- DO NOT allow the patient to walk.
- Handle the patient gently.
- In an incomplete abortion, the physician may direct you to gently attempt removal of the retained products of conception to slow hemorrhage and to relieve or prevent sepsis.

continued

ECTOPIC OR OVARIAN CYST

SIGNS AND SYMPTOMS

1. Abdominal pain and distension
2. Occurs early in pregnancy
3. Missed period
4. Spotting
5. Urge to defecate
6. Referred pain
7. Shock syndrome

TREATMENT

- Multiple large IV's
- Draw blood for type and cross.
- MAST
- O_2

PLACENTA PREVIA

SIGNS AND SYMPTOMS

1. Third trimester
2. Painless vaginal bleeding after or with contractions
3. History of earlier vaginal bleeding
4. Uterus soft, not tender

TREATMENT

- Never perform an internal exam.
- Multiple large IV's/NS. Draw blood for lab work.
- Place the patient on the left side (due to possible supine hypotension syndrome).
- O_2 Max
- MAST (legs only)

ABRUPTIO PLACENTA

SIGNS AND SYMPTOMS

1. Third trimester
2. Severe pain
3. Occasional external blood (most bleeding is internal)
4. Shock syndrome
5. Rigid uterus

TREATMENT

- Treat as for placenta previa.

continued

RUPTURED UTERUS

SIGNS AND SYMPTOMS

1. Tearing sensation
2. Nausea and vomiting/cramping
3. Hard uterus
4. Shock syndrome

HISTORY

- C-sectioned
- Uterine surgery
- Many pregnancies
- Large babies

TREATMENT

Treat as for placenta previa.

ECLAMPSIA/PRE-ECLAMPSIA

SIGNS AND SYMPTOMS

1. Greater than 20 weeks pregnant
2. Usually young patient
3. Edematous
4. Pale
5. Obese
6. Hyperactive
7. Severe cases
   - Headache
   - Vision difficulty
   - Epigastric pain
   - Anxiety
   - Seizures

TREATMENT

- O_2
- IV, D_5W
- Place the patient on the left side.
- Anticipate and control seizures. (Magnesium sulfate is the preferred drug, but valium may be ordered.)
- Transport routine; avoid excitation

DRUG/WEIGHT TABLE FOR PEDIATRIC PATIENTS

Age Avg	Wt Kg	Atropine 1mg/10ml	Benadryl	Calcium Cl 1gm/10ml	Defib	Dextrose 50%	Epinephrine 1mg/10ml	Lidocaine 100mg/5ml	Morphine 1mg/ml	Narcan 0.4/ml	Sodium Bicarb 50meq	Valium 5mg/ml	ET Tube	Vital Signs
		0.01mg/kg	1-2mg/kg	20mg/kg	1-2Joules/kg	1ml/kg	0.01mg/kg 1:10,000	1mg/kg	0.1mg/kg	0.01mg/kg	1meq/kg	0.1-2mg/kg	Premature 3.0	P 140
Neo.	3	0.03mg 0.3cc	3-6mg	60mg 0.6cc	3-6J	3cc	0.03mg 0.3cc	3mg 0.15cc	0.3mg 0.3cc	0.03mg 0.3cc*	3meq 3cc	—	3.5	P 120
	5	0.05mg 0.5cc	5-10mg	100mg 1cc	5-10J	5cc	0.05mg 0.5cc	5mg 0.25cc	0.5mg 0.5cc	0.05mg 0.5cc*	5meq 5cc	—		
6 mo.	6	0.06mg 0.6cc	6-12mg	120mg 1.2cc	6-12J	6cc	0.06mg 0.6cc	6mg 0.3cc	0.6mg 0.6cc	0.06mg 0.6cc*	6meq 6cc	0.6mg 0.12cc	3.5-4.5	P 120. BP 90/60
1 yr.	10	0.1mg 1cc	10-20mg	200mg 2cc	10-20J	10cc	0.1mg 1cc	10mg 0.5cc	1mg 1cc	0.1mg 1.1cc*	10meq 10cc	1mg 0.2cc	4-5.0	P 120. BP 96/54
2 yr.	11	0.11mg 1.1cc	10-20mg	220mg 2.2cc	10-20J	11cc	0.11mg 1.1cc	11mg 0.55cc	1.1mg 1.1cc	0.11mg 1.1cc*	11meq 11cc	1.1mg 0.22cc	5.5	P 110. BP 94/60
3 yr.	15	0.15mg 1.5cc	15-30mg	300mg 3cc	15-30J	15cc	0.15mg 1.5cc	15mg 0.7cc	1.5mg 1.5cc	0.15mg 0.37cc	15meq 15cc	1.5mg 0.3cc	5.5	P 110. BP 100/65
5 yr.	18	0.18mg 1.8cc	20-40mg	360mg 3.6cc	15-30J	18cc	0.18mg 1.8cc	18mg 0.9cc	1.8mg 1.8cc	0.18mg 0.43cc	18meq 18cc	1.8mg 0.35cc	6.0	P 100. BP 94/54
	20	.20mg 2cc	20-40mg	400mg 4cc	20-40J	20cc	0.20mg 2cc	20mg 1cc	2mg 2cc	0.20mg 0.46cc	20meq 20cc	2mg 0.4cc		
7 yr.	22	0.22mg 2.2cc	20-40mg	440mg 4.4cc	20-40J	22cc	0.22mg 2.2cc	22mg 1.1cc	2.2mg 2.2cc	0.22mg 0.5cc*	22meq 22cc	2.2mg 0.45cc	6.5	P 90. BP 102/56
	25	0.25mg 2.5cc	25-50mg	500mg 5cc	25-50J	25cc	0.25mg 2.5cc	25mg 1.2cc	2.5mg 2.5cc	0.25mg 0.6cc	25meq 25cc	2.5mg 0.5cc		
10 yr.	30	0.30mg 3cc	30-60mg	500mg 5cc	30-60J	30cc	0.3mg 3cc	30mg 1.5cc	3mg 3cc	0.3mg 0.75cc	30meq 30cc	3mg 0.6cc	7.0	P 90. BP 110/58
	35	0.35mg 3.5cc	35-70mg	500mg 5cc	35-70J	35cc	0.3mg 3cc	35mg 1.7cc	3.5mg 3.5cc	0.35mg 0.77cc	35meq 35cc	3.5mg 0.7cc		
	40	0.40mg 4cc	40-80mg	500mg 5cc	40-80J	40cc	0.3mg 3cc	40mg 2cc	4.0mg 4.0cc	0.4mg 1cc	40meq 40cc	4mg 0.8cc		
13 yr.	45	0.45mg 4.5cc	45-90mg	500mg 5cc	50-100J	45cc	0.3mg 3cc	45mg 2.2cc	4.5mg 4.5cc	0.4mg 1cc	45meq 45cc	4.5mg 0.9cc	7.5	P 85. BP 114/70

* Mix 0.25cc Narcan and 0.75cc NS, then give indicated dose.

PEDIATRIC ARREST (COR-ZERO) FLOW CHART

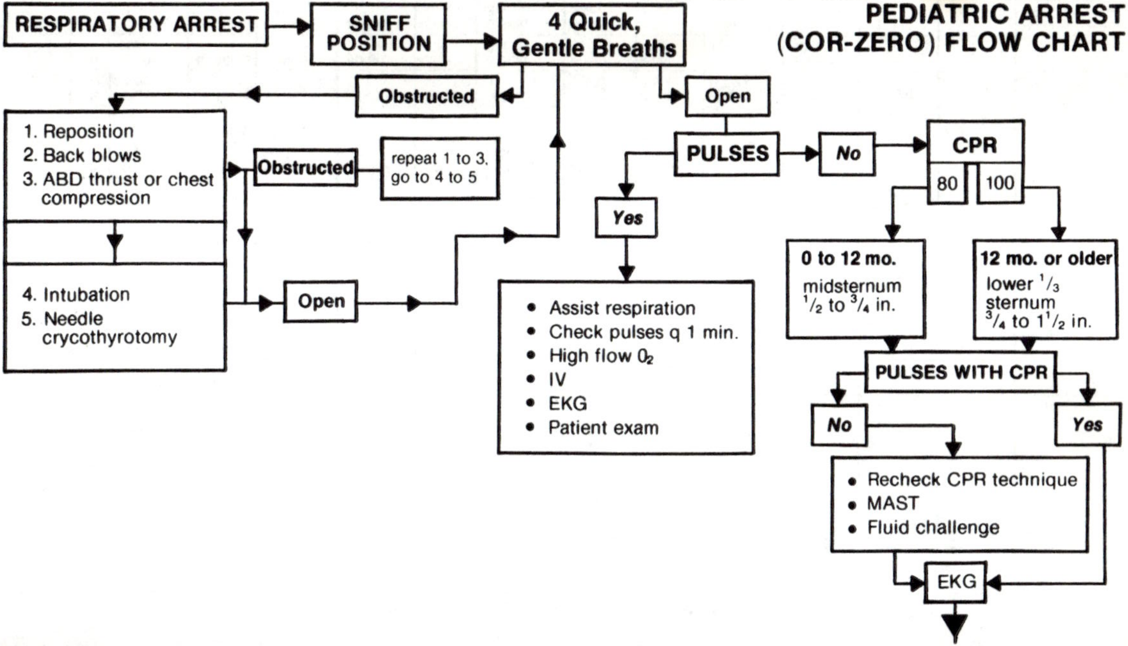

Asystole	Bradycardia	Electromechanical Dissociation	Ventricular Tachycardia	Ventricular Fibrillation
O_2	O_2	O_2	IV-100cc bag	Defib
IV-100cc bag	IV-100cc bag	IV 100cc bag	LIDOCAINE	Treat arrhythmias
BICARB	BICARB	BICARB	Treat arrhythmias	O_2
EPI	ATROPINE	Intubate	O_2-intubate	IV-100cc bag
Intubate	ISOPROTERINOL	EPI	BICARB	BICARB
ATROPINE	________	CALCIUM	________	EPI
ISOPROTERINOL	________	________	________	Defib
CALCIUM	________	________	________	LIDOCAINE
________	________	________	________	________
________	________	________	________	________
________	________	________	________	________
________	________	________	________	________
________	________	________	________	________

LIST DRUG DOSAGES HERE **SEE:** DRUG/WEIGHT TABLE

ATROPINE ________ EPINEPHRINE ________ DEFIB ________

BICARB ________ ISOPROTERINOL ________ CARDIOVERT ________

CALCIUM ________ LIDOCAINE ________

PART SIX
Medications and Procedure Protocols

Aminophylline
Atropine
Bretylium Tosylate (Bretylol)
Calcium Chloride
Dexamethasone (Decadron, Hexadol)
Dextrose 50%
Diazepam (Valium)
Digoxin (Lanoxin)
Diphenhydramine (Benadryl)
Dopamine (Intropin)
Epinephrine (Adrenaline)
Furosemide (Lasix)
Glucagon
Ipecac syrup
Isoproterinol (Isuprel)
IV drip rate table
Lidocaine (Xylocaine, Lidopen)
Mannitol 25% (MSD)
Meperidine (Demorol)
Metaraminol (Aramine)
Morphine Sulfate
Naloxone Hydrochloride (Narcan)
Nitroglycerine (Nitrostat)
Oxygen
Oxytocin (Pitocin)
Phenobarbital (Eskabarb, Luminal Sodium)
Phenytoin Sodium (Dilantin)
Racemic Epinephrine (Vaponephrine)
Sodium Bicarbonate

Crycothyrotomy
Intracardiac Injections
MAST suit
Nasogastric Tube
Nasotracheal Intubation
Pericardiocentesis

AMINOPHYLLINE

By: ☐ **Physician order**
☐ **Protocol** ______________________________
____

DOSAGE

- Adult:
  - 250 to 500mg or 5.6mg/kg in 100cc D_5W IV (piggy-back). Give over 20 min. exactly.
- Ped:
  - 3.5mg/kg in fluid, not to exceed 5ml/kg/hr. (use volume controller). Give over 20 min. exactly.

(Decrease dosage to 1mg/kg if patient is on aminophylline drug or has CHF.)

Local Variance ______________________________

ACTIONS

CNS stimulant; smooth muscle relaxant, including the coronary and bronchial arteries; diuretic effect; decreases peripheral resistance and increases myocardial contraction

INDICATIONS

- Status asthmaticus
- Asthma
- Pulmonary edema from CHF with hypertension
- Emphysema
- Chronic or acute bronchitis

CONTRAINDICATIONS

- When cardiac stimulation would be harmful
- Angina
- Coronary artery disease
- Peptic ulcers
- Glaucoma
- Hypotension
- Hypersensitivity to aminophylline or related drugs

continued

WARNINGS

- DO NOT use if crystals are present.
- Solution should be at room temperature.

ADVERSE REACTIONS

- Headache
- Flushing
- Precordial pain
- Palpitations
- Arrhythmias
- Dizziness
- Hypotension

SIGNS OF INTOXICATION

Restlessness, excitation/drowsiness, tachycardia, arrhythmias, tinnitus, nausea, vomiting, hematemesis and seizures

Note:

FATALITIES ARE USUALLY DUE TO LARGE DOSES IN PATIENTS WITH A HISTORY OF CARDIAC OR RENAL PROBLEMS, OR COPD PATIENTS WHO HAVE SEIZURES SECONDARY TO LARGE DOSES ADMINISTERED TOO RAPIDLY.

ATROPINE

By: ☐ **Physician order**
☐ **Protocol** ______________________

____

DOSAGE

- Adult:
  - 0.5 to 1 mg IV, ET given over 1 min. q 3 to 5 min. to Max of 2 mg
- Ped:
  - 0.01mg/kg as above to Max of two doses

(Use with caution in patients with COPD as it may cause drying of bronchial secretions, causing mucous plugs. For poisonings, 2 to 3mg may be ordered.)

Local Variance ______________________

ACTIONS

Anticholinergic (parasympathetic blocker) that also blocks the actions of other acetylcholine type drugs (increases heart rate by inhibiting vagal tone)

INDICATIONS

- Symptomatic sinus bradycardia
- A/V block
- Sinus block or arrest
- Slow ventricular rates
- Organophosphate poisonings

CONTRAINDICATIONS

- Glaucoma
- Atrial fibrillation
- Tachycardias

ADVERSE REACTIONS

- Dry mouth
- Blurred vision
- Tachycardia
- Photophobia
- Hyperpyrexia
- Dilated pupils

SIGNS OF INTOXICATION

Hot dry skin, thirst, dilated pupils, arrhythmias, excitation, hallucinations, coma, declining Bp and respiratory failure

BRETYLIUM TOSYLATE (Bretylol) *

By: ☐ **Physician order**
☐ **Protocol** ____________________

____

DOSAGE

5mg/kg—If without results, may increase 10mg/kg q 15 to 30 min. Max 30mg/kg, IV PUSH (A drip of 1gm/250cc D W at 1 to 4 mg/min. may be ordered if bretylium caused conversion.)

Local Variance ____________________

ACTIONS

Inhibits norepinephrine release; increases ventricular fibrillation threshold; increases action potential in injured myocardium cells; increases sinoatrial node activity

INDICATIONS

- V-tachycardia
- V-fibrillation

CONTRAINDICATIONS

- None in lethal or potentially lethal arrhythmias

WARNINGS

- Use with caution on digitalis patients.
- 20 min. to 2 hr. onset of action (appears to act in minutes in ventricular fibrillation)

Note:
DO NOT use digitalis and bretylium concurrently.

CALCIUM CHLORIDE 10%

By: ☐ **Physician order**
☐ **Protocol** ______________________

____

DOSAGE

- Adult:
  - 250 to 500mg IV q 10 min.
- Ped:
  - 20mg/kg = 0.2cc/kg

Local Variance ______________________

INDICATIONS

- Asystole
- EMD
- V-fibrillation

CONTRAINDICATIONS

- Coarse V-fibrillation
- Digitalis intoxication

WARNINGS

- Use with caution in patients taking digitalis. Rapid infusion may cause asystole or sinus bradycardia.

ADVERSE REACTIONS

- Hypercalcemia
- Cardiac calcium rigor
- Cardiac arrest

DEXAMETHASONE (Decadron, Hexadol) *

By: ☐ **Physician order**
☐ **Protocol** ______________________

____

DOSAGE

10mg IV

Local Variance ______________________

ACTIONS

Anti-inflammatory

INDICATIONS

- Spinal trauma
- Cerebral edema (from CVA, trauma, tumor or post-cardiac arrest)
- Anaphylactic shock
- Aspiration pneumonia

CONTRAINDICATIONS

- Hypersensitivity to dexamethasone or related drugs

ADVERSE REACTIONS

- Hypertension
- Congestive heart failure in susceptible patients
- Headache
- Vertigo
- Seizures
- Nausea
- Malaise
- Increased insulin reactions in diabetics

SIGNS OF INTOXICATION

A single 10mg dose will probably not show signs of intoxication.

✱ DEXTROSE 50%

By: ☐ **Physician order**
☐ **Protocol** ______________________

____

DOSAGE

- Adult:
  - 50cc s (25gm) IV
- Ped:
  - 1cc/kg IV, diluted 1:1

(Inject over two minutes. Rapid injection may cause thrombosis or embolism.)

Local Variance ______________________

ACTIONS

Increases blood glucose levels. Osmotic diuretic.
Some reports indicate that dextrose 50% may lower the likelihood of stone heart syndrome and provide extra energy for the heart in cardiac arrest situations.

INDICATIONS

- Insulin shock
- Coma from unknown causes or multiple trauma
- Cardiac arrest

WARNINGS

- CHECK FREQUENTLY. Infiltration will cause necrosis of tissue. If infiltration occurs, inject area with 5 to 10cc of lidocaine or NS sub-Q.
- Prior to administration of dextrose 50%, draw and hold blood for lab work.

ADVERSE REACTIONS

- Hyperglycemia

DIAZEPAM (Valium) ✱

By: ☐ **Physician order**
☐ **Protocol** ______________________

____

DOSAGE

- Adult:
  - 2 to 10mg slow IV
- Ped:
  - 0.1mg/kg Max 3 mg IV (not for children under 6 months)

Local Variance ______________________

ACTIONS

Tranquilizer, smooth muscle relaxant and anticonvulsant

INDICATIONS

- Status seizures
- Symptomatic relief in acute alcohol withdrawal
- Prior to cardioversion in conscious/symptomatic arrhythmia patient

CONTRAINDICATIONS

- Hypersensitivity to diazepam or related drugs
- Children under 6 months of age
- Respiratory distressed patients

WARNINGS

- DO NOT mix diazepam with ANY drug.

continued

✱ DIAZEPAM (Valium)

ADVERSE REACTIONS

- Drowsiness
- Confusion
- Amnesia
- Headache
- Nausea
- Tremor
- Altered vision
- Paradoxically:
  - Hyperexcitation
  - Anxiety
  - Hallucinations
  - Rage
  - Increased muscle spasticity

SIGNS OF INTOXCATION

Confusion, somnolence, coma, hypotension, decreased/ absent respirations

- Treatment
  - Airway, O_2, BVM
  - Support respiratory rate.
  - Support Bp with vasopressor.

DIGOXIN (Lanoxin) *

By: ☐ **Physican order**
☐ **Protocol** ______________________

____

DOSAGE

- Adults and children over 10 yrs.
  - 0.45 to 0.6mg slow IV, IM (very painful—use only if unable to give IV)
  - 8 to 12ug/kg in NSR, CHF
  - 10 to 15ug/kg in atrial flutter/fibrillation

(Decrease doses to 6 to 10ug/kg in patients with renal insufficiency. Decrease dose in patients with hypokalemia or hypercalcemia, in patients taking quinidine, or in the very elderly.)

Local Variance ______________________

ACTIONS

Slows AV node conduction; increases myocardial contractions; affects SA node through sympathetic and parasympathetic actions

INDICATIONS

- CHF
- Atrial flutter
- Atrial fibrillation
- PAT

CONTRAINDICATIONS

- V-fibrillation
- Hypersensitivity to digoxin or related drugs
- Possibility of digitalis intoxication

continued

DIGOXIN (Lanoxin)

WARNINGS

- Monitor the patient continually; patients with carditis from rheumatic fever or viral myocarditis,AMI or CHF have marked sensitivity to digoxin induced arrhythmias.
- Use with caution in patients with hypokalemia.
- Digoxin may worsen SA block, or incomplete block.
- Digoxin may increase the rate of W-P-W syndrome.

ADVERSE REACTIONS

- Nausea or vomiting
- Blurred or yellow vision
- Arrhythmias: PVC's, begeminy, group beating, PAT, AV-disassociation or unexplained increases in rate
  TREATMENT:
  - Discontinue digoxin
  - ALS as indicated
- Increasing degree of AV-block
- Excess slowing of pulse
- Pediatric patients: Nausea, visual disturbances; PVC's seldom seen; atrial arrhythmias (PAT, PAC's, atrial tachycardia) most common sign of intoxication

DIPHENHYDRAMINE (Benadryl) *

By: ☐ Physician order
☐ Protocol ______________________

____

DOSAGE

- Adult:
  - 25 to 100mg IV, IM (Max 100mg single dose)
- Ped:
  - 1 to 2mg/kg IV or IM (ages 1 to 12)

(Potentiates atropine, alcohol and CNS depressants)

Local Variance ______________________

ACTIONS

Antihistamine

INDICATIONS

- Blood allergic reactions
- Anaphylaxis
- Antidote for adverse reactions to phenothiazine
- Antiemetic
- Antabuse-alcohol reactions

CONTRAINDICATIONS

- COPD
- Asthma
- Glaucoma
- Hypertension
- Pregnancy
- Hypersensitivity to diphenhydramine or related drugs
- Newborn or premature infants
- Nursing mothers

ADVERSE REACTIONS

- Atrial tachycardia/palpitations
- T-wave changes
- Drowsiness/confusion
- Nervousness/restlessness
- Paradoxically, excitation in children
- Dizziness/vertigo
- Blurred, double vision
- Nausea and vomiting
- Decreased respiratory rates

✱ DOPAMINE HCl (Intropin)

By: ☐ **Physician order**
☐ **Protocol** ______________________________
____

DOSAGE

IV-See charts OR:

- Initially 2 to 5ug/kg/min. (the patient's kg weight × 15 is the number of milligrams to be added to 250cc D_5W. MICRODROP rate equals ug/kg/min.—i.e. 10 microdrops (mcgtts) = 10ug/kg/min.)

(Dosages in patients on MAO inhibitor drugs is 1/10 of normal.)

Local Variance ______________________________

ACTIONS

A Beta action increases myocardial contraction and an Alpha action constricts peripheral vessels. A dopaminergic action increases renal and mesenteric blood flow.

INDICATIONS

- Shock syndromes from:
  - CHF with hypotension
  - AMI
  - Sepsis
  - Renal failure
  - Cardiac failure

CONTRAINDICATIONS

- Hemorrhagic hypotension
- Hypotension from uncorrected tachyarrhythmias or V-fibrillation

WARNINGS

- Monitor Bp closely.
- Extravasation
  - Use large vein if possible. If extravasation occurs, prevent necrosis and sloughing by infiltrating the area as soon as possible with 10 to 15cc of saline solution with 5 to 10mg of phentolamine.

continued

ADVERSE REACTIONS

- Hypotension } Decrease dose!
- Narrowing of pulse pressure }
- Vasoconstriction
  - Occlusive vascular disease—Patient with a history of occlusive vascular disease (for example, atherosclerosis, arterial embolism, Raynaud's disease, cold injury, diabetic endarteritis, and Buerger's disease) should be closely monitored for any changes in color or temperature of the skin in the extremities. If a change in skin color or temperature occurs and is thought to be the result of compromised circulation to the extremities, the benefits of continued dopamine infusion should be weighted against the risk of possible necrosis. This condition may be reversed by either decreasing or discontinuing the rate of infusion.
- Nausea and vomiting
- Headache
- Tachycardia/bradycardia
- Palpitations/angina
- Dyspnea

For a concentration of 1600 mcg Dopamine HCl/ml(4 to 5 ml ampules Intropin/500 ml or 2 to 5 ml ampules Intropin/250 ml)

Body lbs	77	88	99	110	121	132	143	154	165	176	187	198	209	220	231	242
weight kgs	35	40	45	50	55	60	65	70	75	80	85	90	95	100	105	110
FLOW RATE IN DROPS * PER MINUTE																
5	3.8	3.4	2.9	2.6	2.4	2.2	2.0	1.9	1.8	1.6	1.55	1.5	1.4	1.3	1.25	1.2
10	7.6	6.7	5.9	5.3	4.9	4.5	4.1	3.8	3.6	3.3	3.1	3.0	2.8	2.7	2.5	2.4
15	11	10	8.9	8.0	7.3	6.6	6.1	5.7	5.3	5.0	4.7	4.4	4.2	4.0	3.8	3.6
20	15	13	12	11	9.7	8.9	8.2	7.6	7.1	6.7	6.3	5.9	5.6	5.3	5.1	4.9
25	19	17	15	13	12	11	10	9.5	8.9	8.4	7.8	7.4	7.0	6.6	6.3	6.0
30	23	20	18	16	15	13	12	11	11	10	9.4	8.9	8.4	8.0	7.6	7.3
35	27	23	21	19	17	16	14	13	12	12	11	10	9.8	9.3	8.9	8.5
40	31	27	24	21	19	18	16	15	14	13	13	12	11	11	10	9.7
45	34	30	27	24	22	20	18	17	16	15	14	13	13	12	11	11
50	38	33	30	27	24	22	21	19	18	17	16	15	14	13	13	12
55	42	37	33	29	27	24	23	21	20	18	17	16	15	15	14	13
60	46	40	36	32	29	27	25	23	21	20	19	18	17	16	15	15
70	53	47	42	37	34	31	29	27	25	23	22	21	20	19	18	17
80	61	53	47	43	39	36	33	31	28	27	25	24	23	21	20	19
90	69	60	53	48	44	40	37	34	32	30	28	27	25	24	23	22
100	76	67	59	53	49	45	41	38	36	33	31	30	28	27	25	24

DOSAGE = mcg DOPAMINE HCl/kg/min.

* Based on a microdrip calibration of 60 drops equal to 1.0 milliliter.

Note: All dosages of 10 mcg/kg/min. and above have been rounded off to the nearest mcg/kg/min.

Dopamine HCl [Intropin] Effects

The Effects of Intropin at Three Ranges:	2 to 5mcg/ kg/min.	5 to 20mcg/ kg/min.	Over 20mcg/ kg/min.
Cardiac output	no change	increase	increase
Stroke Volume	no change	increase	increase
Heart Rate	no change	There is an initial increase followed by a decrease toward normal rates as infusion continues	
Myocardial Contractility	no change	increase	increase
Potential for Excessive Myocardial Oxygen Demands	low§ coronary blood flow increased	low§ coronary blood flow increased	data unavailable
Potential for Tachyarrhythmias	low§	low§	moderate
Total Systemic Vascular Resistance	slight decrease to no change	no change to slight increase	increase
Renal Blood Flow	increase	increase	decrease
Urine output	increase	increase	decrease

§ Low, but should be monitored.

✱ EPINEPHRINE (Adrenalin)

By: ☐ **Physician order**
☐ **Protocol** ______________________

____

DOSAGE

Arrest (1:10,000)

- Adult:
  - 3 to 5cc (0.3 to 0.5mg) IV - ET q 5 min.
- Ped:
  - 0.1ml/kg (0.01mg/kg) IV - ET q 5 min. Max single dose 0.3mg

Allergic Reactions (1:1,000)

- Adult:
  - 0.3 to 0.5cc (mg) sub-Q
- Ped:
  - 0.005 to 0.3cc (mg) Max 0.3 mg PRN × 3 sub-Q

(Monitor vital signs and cardiac rhythm.)

Local Variance ______________________

ACTIONS

Sympathomimetic—Alpha and Beta stimulation increases myocardial contraction and rate, and decreases bronchoconstriction.

INDICATIONS

- Fine V-fibrillation
- Asystole
- EMD
- Anaphylactic reactions

CONTRAINDICATIONS

- V-tachycardia
- Coarse V-fibrillation

continued

WARNINGS

- DO NOT use if discolored.
- Use caution if pulse is greater than 100, or if patient is older than 40 or is hypotensive.

ADVERSE REACTIONS

- Tachycardia
- Cardiac irritability (monitor patient)
- Arrhythmias
- Cerebrovascular accident (CVA)
- Worsening of angina pain, or may cause onset of pain
- Headache
- Dizziness
- Pallor
- Pupil dilation

✱ FUROSEMIDE (Lasix)

By: ☐ **Physician order**
☐ **Protocol** ____________________

____

DOSAGE

- Adult:
  - 20 to 40mg slow IV or IM. Repeat in 1 to 1½ hrs. if indicated.
- Ped:
  - 1mg/kg IV, IM. Not to exceed adult dose. DO NOT repeat in less than 2 hrs. Give slowly, under close supervision.

Local Variance ____________________

ACTIONS

Diuretic action by inhibiting reabsorption of sodium

INDICATIONS

- Acute pulmonary edema

CONTRAINDICATIONS

- Pregnancy
- Renal failure
- Bladder obstruction
- Hypersensitivity to furosemide or related drugs

WARNINGS

- Use with caution in patients with allergies to sulfa or with a history of cirrhosis.

ADVERSE REACTIONS

- Nausea and vomiting
- Gastric irritation
- Rash or flushing
- Orthostatic hypotension
- Thrombosis or embolism
- Blurred vision
- Tinnitus and hearing loss

Note:

A Foley catheter is indicated if transport will take longer than 15 minutes and patient is comatose.

GLUCAGON *

By: ☐ **Physician order**
☐ **Protocol** ______________________

____

DOSAGE

0.5 to 1mg IV, IM. Repeat if without results in 20 min.

Local Variance ______________________

ACTIONS

Releases glucose stored in the liver; counters bradycardia from propranolol

INDICATIONS

- Insulin shock when unable to establish an IV
- Bradycardia from propranolol O.D.

CONTRAINDICATIONS

- Hypersensitivity to glucagon or related drugs

WARNINGS

- In insulinoma patients, glucagon will initially produce increased glucose levels; but it may cause delayed hypoglycemia due to its insulin-releasing effects.

ADVERSE REACTIONS

- Nausea and vomiting

✱ IPECAC SYRUP

By: ☐ **Physican order**
☐ **Protocol** ______________________

____

DOSAGE

- Adult:
  - 30cc oral, followed by as much water as patient will drink (2 to 3 glasses minimum.). Repeat if no emesis in 20 min.
- Ped:
  - 15cc oral. Give juice or pop first, then follow with water. Repeat if no emesis in 20 min.

Local Variance ______________________

ACTIONS

Gastric irritant that also stimulates the vomiting center in the brain

INDICATIONS

- Emetic

CONTRAINDICATIONS

- Unconscious patients, or those who are lethargic
- Pregnant women/lactating mothers
- Ingestion of strong corrosives
- Strychnine ingestion
- Petroleum distillate injection

WARNINGS

- DO NOT give extract of ipecac as ipecac syrup. If the patient has ingested an antiemetic, ipecac may be ineffective. A second dose should not be given.

ADVERSE REACTIONS

(Although extremely rare, adverse reactions may occur when ipecac syrup has been absorbed, but has not caused emesis.)

- Cardiac conduction disturbances
- Atrial fibrillation
- Fatal myocarditis

ISOPROTERINOL (Isuprel) *

By: ☐ Physician order
☐ Protocol ______________________

____

DOSAGE

- Adult:
  - 1mg in 250cc D_5W IV, piggy-back (4mcg/ml) Start at 1mcg/min. Titrate to pulse of 60 to 80.
- Ped:
  - 1mg in 250cc D_5W (0.07mcg/kg/min. or 1mcg/min., whichever is less). Titrate to pulse of 60 to 80.

mcg/min	mcgtts/min
0.3	5
0.6	10
1	15
1.3	20
2	30
3	45
4	60

(Based on 1 mg in 250cc)

Local Variance ______________________

ACTIONS

Sympathomimetic Beta drug: increases myocardiac contraction and rate; decreases smooth muscle tone

INDICATIONS

- Asystole
- Slow ventricular rates, not affected by atropine

CONTRAINDICATIONS

- Digitalis induced tachycardia

WARNINGS

- Use with caution in patients taking digitalis.
- DO NOT use simultaneously with epinephrine.

continued

✱ ISOPROTERINOL (Isuprel)

ADVERSE REACTIONS

- Increased myocardial oxygen consumption
- Angina
- Arrhythmias
- Nausea and vomiting
- Headache

Note:

Isoproterinol will be less effective in patients taking inderal (Propranolol).

IV DRIP RATE

Drip Rate (cc/hr.)	drops/cc 60	20	15	10
5	5			
10	10	3		
20	20	6	5	3
25	25	8	6	4
30	30	10	8	5
35	35	12	9	6
40	40	13	10	7
45	45	15	11	8
50	50	17	13	9
60	60	20	16	10
75	75	25	19	13
100	100	33	25	17
200	200	66	50	34
300	300	100	75	50
300	300	100	75	50
400	400	133	100	68
500		166	125	84

To use: If 250cc/hr. is ordered using a 10 drop/cc tubing, find the values for 200 and 50 in the 10 column and add these numbers for the drip rate (34+9=43).

-OR-

$$\frac{\text{Total Volume Infused x Drop factor}}{\text{Total Time (in minutes)}} = \text{Drip Rate}$$

-OR-

Number of cc/hr. ÷ Tubing Factor = Drip Rate

Tubing Factor	drops/cc
1	60
4	15
6	10
3	20

✱ LIDOCAINE (Xylocaine, Lidopen)

By: ☐ **Physican order**
☐ **Protocol** ______________________

____

DOSAGE

- Adult:
  - 1mg/kg IV, bolus; Max 300mg
  - After 200mg start drip 1gm/250cc D_5W = 4 mg/ml; Max 4mg/min
- Ped:
  - 1mg/kg IV (no drip in children)
    SEE TABLE NEXT PAGE

Local Variance ______________________

ACTIONS

Increases cell stimulation threshold (decreases ventricular irritability)

INDICATIONS

- PVC's
- V-tachycardia
- V-fibrillation unrefractory to epinephrine
- After defibrillated patient regains pulses

CONTRAINDICATIONS

- 3° AV blocks
- Stokes-Adams syndrome
- Heart blocks
- Hypersensitivity to lidocaine or related drugs

WARNINGS

- Use lidocaine with caution in patients with a history of renal or liver disease.
- Decrease the dosage if there is a history of respiratory depression.

continued

ADVERSE REACTIONS

- CNS depression or stimulation
- Seizures
- Hypotension
- Respiratory arrest
- Bradycardia

SIGNS OF INTOXICATION

Prolongation of the PR interval and QRS complex, or arrhythmias/seizures should indicate decreasing the drip rate.

mg/min	mcgtts/min
1	15
2	30
3	45
4	60

(Based on 1 gm in 250cc)

✱ MANNITOL 25% (MSD)

By: ☐ **Physician order**
☐ **Protocol** ______________________________

____

DOSAGE

- Adult:
  - 1 to 2gm/kg IV over 30 to 60 min. through filtered IV set
- Ped:
  - (Dosages in children under 12 are not established. Monitor cardiovascular/pulmonary status closely. Increased extracellular fluid may cause pulmonary edema or congestive failure.)

Local Variance ______________________________

ACTIONS

Osmotic diuretic

INDICATIONS

- Cerebral edema without signs of active cerebral bleeding

CONTRAINDICATIONS

- Renal disease (severe)
- Pulmonary edema
- Severe dehydration
- Active intracranial bleeding
- Pregnancy

continued

WARNINGS

- Insert a Foley catheter.
- DO NOT use mannitol 25% if crystals are present (always use filtered administration set).

ADVERSE REACTIONS

- Pulmonary edema
- Electrolyte imbalances
- Nausea and vomiting/diarrhea
- Headache
- Blurred vision
- Seizures
- Tachycardia
- Anginalike chest pain
- Hyper/hypotension
- Thrombophlebitis
- Arm pain

✱ MEPERIDINE (Demerol)

By: ☐ **Physician order**
☐ **Protocol** ______________________________

____

DOSAGE

- Adult:
  - 50 to 100mg q 3 to 4 hrs. IM sub-Q
- Ped:
  - 1mg/kg q 3 to 4 hrs. IM sub-Q

(May also be given ½ IV, ½ IM. Administer slowly; have narcan and respiratory support ready. Use with great caution in patients taking other narcotics, sedatives, tranquilizers or antidepressants.)

Local Variance ______________________________

ACTIONS

Narcotic analgesic similar to morphine (has more rapid onset and shorter duration than morphine)

INDICATIONS

- Control of severe pain

CONTRAINDICATIONS

- Hypersensitivity to meperidine or related drugs
- Head injuries
- Abdominal pain
- Pregnancy and nursing mothers
- Atrial-fibrillation/supraventricular tachycardia (relative contraindication)

continued

MEPERIDINE (Demerol)

WARNINGS

- Use a decreased dosage in elderly and those with COPD, asthma, or seizure disorders.

ADVERSE REACTIONS

- Nausea and vomiting
- Dizziness
- Confusion
- Seizures
- Arrhythmias
- CNS depression
- Dilated pupils
- Respiratory/cardiac arrest
- Pain at injection site
- Localized or general allergic reactions

SIGNS OF INTOXICATION

Respiratory depression/arrest; Cheyne-Stokes; cyanosis; extreme somnolence (stupor/coma); shock syndrome

- Treatment
  - Narcan and ALS as indicated

✱ METARAMINOL (Aramine)

By: ☐ Physician order
☐ Protocol ______________________

____

DOSAGE

100mg in 250cc D_5W IV. Start at 20 to 30mcgtts/min. to BP of 90; increase rate AFTER 10 min. if Bp is not affected. Use with caution in patients with a history of (a) taking digitalis, (b) cirrhosis, (c) thyroid disease, (d) hypertension, (e) heart disease or (f) diabetes.

Local Variance ______________________

ACTIONS

A sympathomimetic amine that increases systolic and diastolic Bp; increased myocardial contraction and peripheral vasoconstriction; may decrease blood flow to vital organs

INDICATIONS

- Neurogenic shock
- Cardiogenic shock
- Septic shock
- Drug reaction induced shock

CONTRAINDICATIONS

- Hypovolemia
- Head injury
- Hypersensitivity to metaraminol or related drugs

continued

METARAMINOL (Aramine) *

WARNINGS

- DO NOT INFILTRATE!
- USE LARGE VEINS.

ADVERSE REACTIONS

- Excess blood pressure elevation
- Secondary complications of excess Bp elevation
  - CVA
  - Pulmonary edema
  - Arrhythmias
  - Cardiac arrest
- Arrhythmias, especially in cardiogenic shock patients
- Relapse of malaria
- Necrosis of infiltrated tissue
- Nausea and vomiting
- Reflex bradycardias

Note:

Check Bp every 5 minutes.

✱ MORPHINE SULFATE (Morphine)

By: ☐ **Physician order**
☐ **Protocol** ____________________

____

DOSAGE

- Adult:
  - 2mg SLOW IV q 5 min. until pain is relieved (Max 5mg IV)
- Ped:
  - 0.01 to 0.02mg/kg sub-Q or SLOW IV

(Have narcan and respiratory support ready.)

Local Variance ____________________

ACTIONS

Analgesic; also depresses cough center and stimulates vomiting

INDICATIONS

- Analgesic in chest pain of AMI origin
- Acute pulmonary edema

CONTRAINDICATIONS

- Hypersensitivity to morphine sulfate or related drugs
- Seizure states
- Pulmonary edema as a result of chemical irritant
- Head injury

continued

WARNINGS

- Use morphine sulfate with caution in patients with a history of diseases characterized by hypothyroidism, hypoxia, and renal or liver disfunction.

ADVERSE REACTIONS

- Dizziness
- Euphoria
- Hypotension
- Nausea and vomiting
- Seizures

SIGNS OF INTOXICATION

Respiratory depression, Cheyne-Stokes, cyanosis, stupor, coma, hypotension, bradycardia, apnea and cardiac arrest

Note:

NALAXONE HYDROCHLORIDE (NARCAN) IS AN ANTIDOTE FOR OVERDOSE.

NALOXONE HYDROCHLORIDE (Narcan)

By: ☐ **Physician order**
☐ **Protocol** ______________________

____

DOSAGE

- Adult:
  - 0.4 to 2mg IV, IM q 2 to 3 min.
- Ped:
  - 0.01mg/kg (administer as per adult)

Local Variance ______________________

ACTIONS

Narcotic antagonist

INDICATIONS

- Narcotic overdose
  - (Effective or partly effective against: codeine, Darvocet, Darvon, Demerol, Dilaudid, heroin, Lomotil, methadone, morphine, Percocet, Percodan and Talwin)
- Coma of unknown causes
- Mixed unknown overdoses

CONTRAINDICATIONS

- Hypersensitivity to nalaxone hydrochloride or related drugs.

WARNINGS

- Use with caution in suspected addicted patients, including newborns. (Watch for recurrence of O.D. signs as nalaxone hydrochloride wears off.)

ADVERSE REACTIONS

Abrupt reversal of narcotic induced depression can cause:

- Nausea and vomiting
- Tachycardia
- Diaphoresis
- Hypertension
- Tremors

NITROGLYCERIN (Nitrostat) *

By: ☐ **Physician order**
☐ **Protocol** ______________________

____

DOSAGE

0.4mg (1/150) sublingual q 5 min. to Max 1.2mg

Local Variance ______________________

ACTIONS

Relaxes smooth muscles (vasodilatory effect)

INDICATIONS

- Angina pectoris
- Pulmonary edema (if Bp is over 120/80)

CONTRAINDICATIONS

- Hypersensitivity to nitroglycerin or related drugs
- Severe anemia
- AMI
- CVA

WARNINGS

- Discontinue use if blurring of vision or drying of mouth occurs.
- Use with caution in patients with glaucoma.
- A vasodilatory effect is more marked in dehydrated persons.

ADVERSE REACTIONS

- Headache (an expected effect)
- Dizziness
- Postural hypotension
- Palpitations
- Blurring of vision
- Drying of mouth

OXYGEN: REMAINING TIME

		Liter Flow Rate									
	TANK SIZE	2	3	4	5	6	7	8	9	10	15
250 PSI	D	20	13	10	8	7	6	5	4.4	4	3
	E	35	23	18	14	12	10	9	8	7	5
	150	238	158	119	95	79	68	59	53	48	32
	G	301	200	150	120	100	86	75	67	60	40
	H-K	393	262	196	157	130	112	98	87	78	52
500 PSI	D	40	27	20	16	13	11	10	9	8	5
	E	70	47	35	28	23	20	17	15	14	9
	150	475	316	237	190	158	135	119	106	95	63
	G	603	402	301	241	200	172	150	133	120	80
	H-K	750	500	375	300	250	215	187	166	150	100
1000 PSI	D	80	53	40	32	26	23	20	18	16	11
	E	140	93	70	56	46	40	35	31	28	19
	150	950	633	475	380	316	271	238	211	190	126
	G	1025	803	602	482	401	344	301	265	241	161
	H-K	1570	1046	785	628	523	448	392	348	314	209

Note:

MAX. FLOW NASAL 10

MIN. MASK 6

Use of table for PSI other than listed:
i.e.—750PSI, D tank, 2 liters
Add 20 (250PSI) + 40 (500PSI) = 60 min.

OXYTOCIN (Pitocin) *

By: ☐ **Physician order**
☐ **Protocol** ______________________________

____

DOSAGE

10 to 40 units in 1000cc NS D_5W LR
Titrate to increased Bp, uterine tone and decreased blood loss.

Local Variance ______________________________

ACTIONS

Increases uterine tone, allowing increased contraction

INDICATIONS

- Control of postpartum uterine bleeding

CONTRAINDICATIONS

- Normal pregnancy
- Vaginal bleeding BEFORE delivery
- Severe toxemia
- Hypersensitivity to oxytocin or related drugs

WARNINGS

- NOT to be given for reinforcement of existing labor

ADVERSE REACTIONS

- Allergic reactions
- Hypotension
- Arrhythmias
- Hypertension
- Hypertonic uterine spasms or contractions

✱ PHENOBARBITAL (Eskabarb, Luminal Sodium)

By: ☐ **Physician order**
☐ **Protocol** ______________________________

____

DOSAGE

- Adult:
  - 200 to 300mg SLOW IV. Titrate to patient response. Give over 5 to 10 min.
- Ped:
  - 3 to 5mg/kg SLOW IV. Titrate to patient response. Give over 5 to 10 min.

Local Variance ______________________________

ACTIONS

Anticonvulsant that decreases the excitability of the central nervous system

INDICATIONS

- Status epilepticus
- Eclampsia

CONTRAINDICATIONS

- Hypersensitivity to phenobarbital or related drugs
- Respiratory distress
- Sub-Q

continued

PHENOBARBITAL (Eskabarb, Luminal Sodium) *

WARNINGS

- Use with caution in nursing mothers (may produce drowsiness in infants).

ADVERSE REACTIONS

- Hypersensitivity reactions
- Thrombophlebitis from IV injection
- CNS depression
- Delirium
- Occasionally, excitation and CNS stimulation
- Systemic pain

SIGNS OF INTOXICATION

Progressive CNS depression, confusion, headache, coma, dizziness, respiratory arrest/depression, shock syndrome, pulmonary edema, hypothermia/hyperpyrexia

- Treatment
  - Supportive: BLS and ALS as indicated

✱ PHENYTOIN SODIUM (Dilantin)

By: ☐ **Physician order**
☐ **Protocol** ______________________

____

DOSAGE

- Adult:
  - 150 to 200mg; not to exceed 50mg/min. IV
- Ped:
  - Not to exceed 25mg/min. IV

(Not recommended in nursing mothers: may affect infant)

Local Variance ______________________

ACTIONS

Inhibits spread of seizure activity across motor cortex; appears to stabilize the cells; hyperexcitability caused by changes in the cell membrane sodium gradient

INDICATIONS

- Control of epileptic seizures

CONTRAINDICATIONS

- Hypersensitivity to phenytoin sodium or related drugs

WARNINGS

Patients with liver disease or who are gravely ill may show early signs of intoxication.

ADVERSE REACTIONS

- Confusion
- Dizziness
- Slurred speech
- Nystagmus
- Nausea and vomiting
- Motor twitching
- Headache
- Nervousness

continued

PHENYTOIN SODIUM (Dilantin) *

SIGNS OF INTOXICATION

- Lethargy
- Slurred speech
- Nystagmus
- Hyperreflexia
- Nausea and vomiting
- Tremors
- Coma
- Hypotension
- Bradycardia
- Arrhythmias

TREATMENT OF INTOXICATION

- Supportive: ALS as indicated

✱ RACEMIC EPINEPHRINE (Vaponephrine)

By: ☐ **Physician order**
☐ **Protocol** ____________________

____

DOSAGE

- Adult - Ped:
  - Inhalation of 1cc diluted with normal saline in nebulizer (8 liter/min of O_2) DO NOT repeat.

(DO NOT use if discolored or if precipitate is present.)

Local Variance ____________________

ACTIONS

Localized epinephrine

INDICATIONS

- Bronchial asthma
- Croup

CONTRAINDICATIONS

- V-tachycardia
- Coarse V-fibrillation

WARNINGS

- Monitor patients closely. Patients with heart disease, hypertension, diabetes or thyroid disease are more susceptible to side effects.

ADVERSE REACTIONS

- Increased pulse
- Increased blood pressure
- Arrhythmias
- Headache
- Anxiety
- Tremors

SODIUM BICARBONATE *

By: ☐ **Physician order**
☐ **Protocol** ______________________

____

DOSAGE

- Adult:
  - 1Meg/kg repeated in 10 min., then half initial dose q 10 min.
- Ped:
  - Same, diluted 1:1 with D_5W. GIVE SLOWLY!

Local Variance ______________________

ACTIONS

Increases blood bicarbonate; reverses acidosis

INDICATIONS

- Cardiac arrest
- Acidosis from profound shock
- Certain poisonings
- Severe diabetic ketoacidosis
- Severe diarrhea

CONTRAINDICATIONS

- Congestive heart failure
- Hypokalemia
- Patients with history of excessive vomiting
- Marked edema

WARNINGS

- Rapid infusion may cause hypernatremia, acidosis, and cerebral or pulmonary edema. Give slowly.

ADVERSE REACTIONS

- Alkalosis (decreases O_2 released to tissue)
- Hyperirritability/tetany

Procedures

Crycothyrotomy
Intracardiac Injections
MAST suit
Nasogastric Tube
Nasotracheal Intubation
Pericardiocentesis

CRYCOTHYROTOMY ✱

By: ☐ Physician order
☐ Protocol ________________________

____

INDICATIONS

- Obstructed airway
- Airway that cannot be maintained by any other means
- Trauma arrests

PROCEDURE: (Adult)

1. Locate the crycothyroid space.
2. Pinch a small area of skin over the crycothyroid and pull it away from the neck. Remove this tissue with scissors. This allows visualization of underlying structures.
3. Stabilize soft tissue and cartilage.
4. With a #10 blade, make a stabbing, transverse entry.
5. Dilate the incision using a gloved little finger, pediatric nasal speculum, otic earpiece or scalpel handle.
6. Pass an ET tube ½ to 1 inch, then inflate the cuff and secure it in place.
7. Check breath sounds. The tube may have gone into the pharynx.

PROCEDURE: (Pediatric)

1. Locate the crycothyroid space.
2. Use a #14 catheter type needle and a syringe.
3. Enter the trachea and check for air using the syringe.
4. Angle the needle toward the feet as soon as the needle passes through the membrane.
5. Pass the catheter and remove the needle.
6. Using an O_2 mask, apply 10 to 15 liters over the area.

CAUTIONS/COMPLICATIONS

- Damge to larynx, vocal cords, esophagus, cartilages
- Bleeding from thyroid, carotid arteries, jugulars, esophagus
- False passage of tube
- Sub-Q air
- Stenosis

✱ INTRACARDIAC INJECTIONS

By: ☐ **Physician order**
☐ **Protocol** ______________________________
____

INDICATIONS

- Cardiac arrest, when unable to establish an IV
- When a direct effect on the heart is desired

PROCEDURE: (Adult)

1. Locate the required landmark(s)
   - ☐ 4th intercostal space 2cm left of sternum at 90°
   - ☐ 5th intercostal space 2cm left of sternum, aiming toward head at 70 to 80° angle
   - ☐ Subxiphoid, immediately below and left of process, aiming toward AC joint at 45° angle
2. Prep the patient's skin.
3. Advance the needle using a sharp, quick thrust under the patient's skin.
4. Aspirate the needle while advancing it.
5. When blood returns freely, inject the medication quickly.
6. Quickly withdraw the needle, pressing an alcohol prep or a 4x4 pad over the site.

PROCEDURE: (Children)

1. Use a 3", #20 gauge needle.
2. Locate landmarks
   - ☐ Subxiphoid, 20° angle toward 3rd intercostal space on the midclavicular line
   - ☐ 3rd intercostal space at 90° straight in
   - ☐ 4th intercostal space toward head at 70 to 80°
3. Proceed to steps 2 through 6 in the adult procedure.

PROCEDURE: (Infant)

1. Locate the subxiphoid landmark only.
2. Use a 1½", #21 gauge needle.
3. Advance the needle at a 20° angle, aiming toward the left midclavicular line.
4. Proceed to steps 2 through 6 in the adult procedure.

CAUTIONS/COMPLICATIONS

- Do not delay CPR longer than needed.
- Pericardial tamponade
- Pneumothorax
- Hemothorax
- Lacerations to the heart or coronary arteries

BY: ☐ Physician order
☐ Protocol ____________________

____

INDICATIONS

- Hypovolemic hypotension with Bp less than 80
- Uninflated on all multitrauma or potential hypovolemic patients
- CPR
- EMD (not all lack of pulses is EMD)
- Uncontrolled bleeding of arterial injuries of the lower extremities
- Major pelvis or lower extremity fractures
- To convert PAT

PROCEDURE:

1. Position the MAST before moving the patient to a cot or long board. Try putting the pants on your arms, then grab the patient by the ankles and pull the pants onto the patient like a pair of trousers. This keeps the straps straight and speeds up application.
2. Inflate the MAST as much as you can with your mouth, then use a pump until the velcro crackles or until the pressure is up to 30 to 40 mmHg.
3. Check for changes in Bp and for signs of respiratory distress.
4. DO NOT deflate the MAST in the field without the physician's orders.

CAUTIONS/COMPLICATIONS

- Respiratory compromise if placed too high
- Pulmonary edema (deflate abdomen if this occurs)
- Emesis, defecation and/or urination can occur due to increased abdominal pressure
- In some situations, inflation of legs only may be indicated (i.e.—advanced pregnancy).

✱ NASOGASTRIC TUBE

By: ☐ Physician order
☐ Protocol ______________________________

____

INDICATIONS

- Distended abdomen in severe abdominal pain
- Distended abdomen in cardiac arrest
- Unconscious, intubated patients with emesis or abdominal trauma

PROCEDURE:

1. Lubricate the tube and instill viscous xylocaine 2% in the largest nostril.
2. Slightly flex the patient's head forward.
3. Insert the tube straight into the nostril (90°).
4. Gently rotate the tube and apply pressure until the tube makes the bend.
5. Advance the tube. (If the patient is conscious, the tube should be swallowed rapidly as it is advanced.)
6. Check for placement by listening for an air bubble while injecting 20 to 30cc of air.
7. Aspirate the gastric contents.
8. Secure the tube.

CAUTIONS/COMPLICATIONS

- Have suction ready.
- The procedure may cause nosebleed.
- Do not force the tube.
- Intracranial placement is possible if the tube is forced in patients with skull fractures. STOP if any resistance is encountered in these patients.

NASOTRACHEAL INTUBATION *

By: ☐ Physician order
☐ Protocol ______________________

____

INDICATIONS

- ANY patient who is breathing and is/or exhibits:
  - Unconscious
  - Low gag reflex
  - Acute chest trauma
  - O.D.
  - Tracheal trauma or burns

PROCEDURE:

1. Have suction ready.
2. Oxygenate the patient prior to attempt.
3. Position the patient supine with the head in a sniff position (no hyperextension or midline rotation).
4. Select the proper tube size (men 8 to 9; women 7 to 8).
5. Select the largest naris.
6. Lubricate the tube and instill lubricant in the nose.
7. From the head of the patient and with the curve of tube opposite normal, pass the tube straight into the nose (90°) until the tube stops. Gently rotate the tube, applying pressure until the tube makes the bend and the tube is in the normal curved position.
8. Pass the tube to the point of maximum sound.
9. Gently displace the trachea posteriorly.
10. Rapidly advance the tube upon inspiration.
11. Check breath sounds bilaterally, then inflate the cuff and secure the tube.

CAUTIONS/COMPLICATIONS

- Gagging
- Vomiting
- Epistaxis
- Intracranial placement in presence of skull fracture
  - Use caution if blood or CSF is present.
  - DO NOT force the tube.
  - You MUST hear breathing through the tube at all times.

✱ PERICARDIOCENTESIS

By: ☐ Physician order
☐ Protocol ______________________

____

INDICATIONS

- Cardiac tamponade
  - Inaudible heart sounds
  - Tachycardia
  - Hypotension
  - Distension of neck veins
  - Paradoxical pulse
  - Narrow pulse pressure
- Trauma arrest with chest injury

PROCEDURE:

1. Locate the proper landmark below the left rib cage and left of the xiphoid process.
2. Prep the patient's skin.
3. Advance the needle at a 45° angle toward the right sternoclavicular joint.
4. Aspirate while inserting the needle 8 to 10cm. (stop when blood returns).
5. Evacuate available blood; change syringes if necessary.
6. Withdraw the needle and apply pressure to the site.

CAUTIONS/COMPLICATIONS

- Lacerations of ventricle or coronary artery
- Pneumothorax
- Hemothorax

PART SEVEN
Emergency References

Abbreviations and Symbols Used in Field Charting
Common Prescription Drug Names and Classifications
Patient Survey
Phone Numbers
Radio Telemetry Code Phone Book

ABBREVIATIONS AND SYMBOLS USED IN FIELD CHARTING

@	at
A.A.	auto accident
AAOX	awake, alert, and oriented times________
AB	abortion
abd	abdomen
adm.	admission
AMA	against medical advice
AMI	acute myocardial infarction
ant.	anterior
AOB	alcohol on board
ASCVD	arteriosclerotic cardiovascular disease
ASHD	arteriosclerotic heart disease
ass't	assisted/assist
a&p	auscultation and percussion
A&P	anterior and posterior
$\approx$	approximately
BBB	bundle branch block
b.i.d.	twice a day
bil.	bilateral
BM	bowel movement
Bp	blood pressure
B.S.	breath sounds
BVM	bag valve mask
Bx	biopsy
$\bar{c}$	with
Ca	cancer
CAB	coronary artery bypass
CAD	coronary artery disease
CAOx	conscious, alert, oriented times (1) person (2) place (3) time
cath.	catheter, catheterization
cc	cubic centimeter
CC:	chief complaint
CCU	coronary care unit
CHF	congestive heart failure
chg. or Δ	change
CHI	closed head injury
cm	centimeter
CNS	central nervous system
CO_2	carbon dioxide

Abbreviations and Symbols (continued)

COLD	chronic obstructive lung disease
COPD	chronic obstructive pulmonary disease
CPR	cardiopulmonary resuscitation
CS	central supply
C-section	Cesarean section
C-spine	cervical spine
CSF	cerebrospinal fluid
CVA	cerebral vascular accident
CVP	central venous pressure
c/o	complains of
detox	detoxification
DOA	dead on arrival
DNR	do not resuscitate
Dr.	doctor
drsg or dsg	dressing
DT	delirium tremens
Dx	diagnosis
d/c	discontinue
D&C	dilatation and curettage
↓	decreased
ea	each
EAO	esophageal obturator airway
ECF	Extended Care Facility
ECG or EKG	electrocardiogram
ED	Emergency Department
EENT	eye, ear, nose, and throat
ENT	ear, nose, and throat
EOM	extraocular movement
ER	emergency room
et	and
ET	endotracheal tube
etc	and so on
ETOH	alcohol
exam	examination
=	equal
F or ♀	female
F.B. and f.b.	foreign body
ft	foot or feet
Fx	fracture
GC	gonococcus or gonorrhea
G.I.	gastrointestinal
gm	gram
gr	grain

Abbreviations and Symbols (continued)

G.S.W.	gun shot wound
gtt	drop
gtts	drops
GU	genitourinary
GYN	gynecology
→	going to or leading to
$>$	greater than
HA	headache
Hct	hematocrit [red blood cells per cc]
Hgb	hemoglobin
h.s.	at bedtime
ht.	height
Hx	history
hypo	hypodermic
H&P	history and physical
H_2O	water
ICU	intensive care unit
IM	intramuscular
inf.	inferior
IV	intravenous
I&D	incision and drainage
I&O	intake and output
↑	increased
K.O.	knocked out
K.V.O.	keep vein open
K+	potassium
l	liter
L	left
lat.	lateral
lb.	pound
LBBB	left bundle branch block
lg.	large
liq.	liquid
LLL	left lower lobe
LLQ	left lower quadrant
LMP	last menstrual period
L.O.C.	loss of consciousness or level of consciousness
L-spine	lumbar spine
lt	left
LUL	left upper lobe
LUQ	left upper quadrant
$<$	less than

Abbreviations and Symbols (continued)

M or ♂	male
mcg	microgram
MCL	midclavicular line
meds	medication
MEq or Meq	milliequivalent
mg	milligram
Mg	magnesium
MI or M.I.	myocardial infarction
misc.	miscellaneous
ml	milliliter
mm	millimeter
MOE	movement of extremities
MS	multiple sclerosis
NaCL or N/S	normal saline
neg. or -	negative
neuro	neurology
N.H.	nursing home
NKA	no known allergies
noc. or noct.	night
NPO	nothing by mouth
NSR	normal sinus rhythm
NT	nasotracheal tube
N&V&D or NV&D	nausea and vomiting and diarrhea
θ	none
OB	obstetrics
o.d.	right eye
O.D.	overdose
O.J.	orange juice
ophth.	ophthalmology
O.R.	operating room
Orth.	orthopedics
os	by mouth
o.s.	left eye
o.u.	both eyes
oz. or ℥	ounce
0_2	oxygen
p	after
PAC	premature atrial contraction
para	number of pregnancies
PAT	paraxysmal atrial tachycardia
path.	pathology
PE	physical examination

Abbreviations and Symbols (continued)

peds	pediatrics
per	by or through
PERLA	pupils equal, react to light/accommodate
PG	pregnant
P.I.	present illness
P.I.D.	pelvic inflammatory disease
PND	paraxysmal nocturnal dyspnea
p.o.	by mouth
post.	posterior
pos or +	positive
pt	patient
P.T.A.	prior to arrival
psych.	psychiatric
PVC	premature ventricular contractions
Px	physical
q	every
q.d.	daily
q.i.d.	four times a day
q.o.d.	every other day
R	right
RBBB	right bundle branch block
resp	respirations
RLQ	right lower quadrant
ROM	range of motion
ROS	review of systems
RSR	regular sinus rhythm
RUQ	right upper quadrant
Rx	prescription
R/O	rule out
$\bar{s}$	without
sm.	small
SOB	shortness of breath
sol.	solution
stat	at once
sub-Q	subcutaneous
sup.	superior
surg.	surgery
S&M	sensation and motion
SM&C	sensation, motion and circulation
2°	secondary or second degree
TAB	therapeutic abortion
TB	tuberculosis

Abbreviations and Symbols (continued)

tbsp.	tablespoon
temp.	temperature
TIA	transient ischemic attack
t.i.d.	three times a day
TKO	to keep open
TLC	tender loving care
TM	tympanic membranes
tol.	tolerated
tsp.	teaspoon
Tx	traction/transport/treatment
∴	therefore
URI	upper respiratory infection
uro	urology
UTI	urinary tract infection
U/A	upon arrival
≠	unequal
vag	vaginal
VD	venereal disease
via	by way of
vol.	volume
V.S.	vital signs
wc	wheelchair
WNL	within normal limits
wt.	weight
x or X	times
yr	year(s)
	lying ⎤ orthostatic vital signs
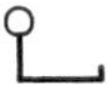	sitting ⎦
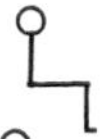	sitting, feet down
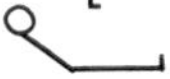	reclining, semi-Fowlers
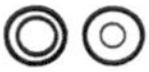	pupils unequal R or L
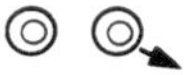	eye/eyes look to arrow
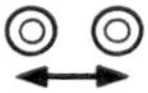	eyes wander

COMMON PRESCRIPTION DRUG NAMES AND CLASSIFICATIONS

1. Analgesic: Acetaminophen and combinations
2. Analgesic: Aspirin and codeine
3. Analgesic: Aspirin and combinations
4. Analgesic: Salicylates and combinations
5. Analgesic: Synthetics, morphine, opium derivatives and combinations
6. Analgesic: Potent synthetics and/or combinations
7. Other analgesics
8. Anorexic—amphetamines
9. Anorexic—nonamphetamines
10. Antiasthmatic
11. Anticoagulant
12. Anticonvulsant
13. Antidepressants
14. Antidiabetic (oral)
15. Cold preparation with narcotics
16. Tranquilizer
17. Quinidine
18. Sedative—Barbiturate
19. Sedative—Nonbarbiturate
20. Muscle relaxant
21. Skeletal muscle relaxant with an analgesic
22. Smooth muscle relaxant
23. Antiarrhythmiac
24. Antihypertensive
25. Antihypertensive with diuretic
26. Digitalis
27. Vasodilator (coronary acting)
28. Tricyclic
29. Antiarrhythmiac (beta blocker)

Drug Names	Classification Number
A.P.C. with Codeine	3, 5, 15
Accurbron	10
Acenocoumarol	11
Actifed-C Expectorant	15
Adapin	13, 16, 28
Adatuss D.C. Expectorant Cough Syrup	5, 6, 15
Adipex-P Tablets	9
Aerolate	27
Aldactazide	24, 25
Aldactone	24
Aldoclor Tablets	25
Aldomet	2
Aldoril Tablets	25
Alurate Elixir	18
Ambenyl Expectorant	15
Amesec	10
AminA 21	9, 13
Aminodur Dura-Tabs	10
Aminophylline	27, 10
Amitad	13, 28
Amitril	13, 28
Amitriptyline Hydrochloride	13, 28
Amoxapine	13, 28
Amytal	18
Amytal Sodium Ampules	12
Anaprox Tablets	7
Anisindione	11
Anorexin Capsules	9
Antabuse	9
Appedrine	9
Apresazide	25
Apresoline-Esidrix	25
Aquaphyllin Syrup and I.R. Capsules	10
Arthralgen	1
Ascriptin with Codeine	5
Asendin	13, 28
Atarax	16
Atenolol	29
Ativan	16, 19
Aventyl	13, 28
Azene Capsules	16
B & O Supprettes No. 15A and No. 16A	5

continued

Drug Names	Classification Number
Bancap Capsules	1
Bancap with Codeine Capsules	5
Bayer Children's Cold Tablets	3
Beclovent Inhaler	10
Benzedrine Spansule Capsules and Tablets	8
Blocadren	29
Bontril PDM	9
Brethine	10
Bretylol	23
Bronkephrine Hydrochloride Injection	10
Bronkodyl	10
Bronkodyl S-R	10
Bronkometer	10
Bronkosol	10
Bronkotabs	10
Buff-A Comp	18, 3
Buticaps	18
Butisol Sodium	18
Calcidrine Syrup	15
Capital with Codeine	1
Capital with Codeine Suspension	5
Capital with Codeine Tablets	5
Carbrital	18
Cardilate	27
Cardioquin	17, 23
Cartrax	27
Catapres	24
Cedilanid-D	26
Celontin	12
Cenadex	9, 16
Choledyl	10
Circubid	22
Clonopin	12
Codalan	5
Codimal DH, PH	15
Colrex	15
Combipres	25
Compazine	16
Comtrex	1
Congespirin	3
Congespirin Liquid Cold Medicine	1
Control Capsules	9

continued

Drug Names	Classification Number
Corgard	24, 29
Coumadin	11
Co-Xan	10
Crystodigin	26
Dalmane	19
Dantrium	20
Darvocet-N	6
Darvon	6
Darvon with A.S.A.	6
Darvon Compound	6
Darvon Compound-65	6
Darvon-N	6
Darvon-N with A.S.A.	6
Datril 500	1
Demerol APAP	6
Demerol Hydrochloride	5
Demi-Regroton	24
Demser Capsules	24
Depakene Capsules and Syrup	12
Deprol	13, 16
Desepramine	28
Desoxyn	8
Dexatrim Capsules	9
Dexedrine	8
Diabinese	14
Dialog	1, 18
Dicodid	5
Dicumarol	11
Didrex Tablets	8
Dilantin	12
Dilaudid Cough Syrup	15
Dilaudid Hydrochloride	5
Dipaxin	11
Diucardin	24
Diulo	24
Diupres	25
Diuril	24
Diutensen Tablets	25
Diutensen-R Tablets	25
Dolophine Hydrochloride Ampules and Vials	5
Dolophine Hydrochloride Tablets	5
Doxepin	28

continued

Drug Names	Classification Number
Duotrate 45	27
Duotrate Plateau	27
Duradyne DHC Tablets	5
Duraquin	23
Dyazide	25
Dymelor	14
Elavil Tablets and Injection	13, 28
Elixicon Suspension	10
Elixophyllin	10
Empirin with Codeine	2
Empracet with Codeine	1
Empracet with Codeine Phosphate No.'s 3 & 4	5
Emprazil Tablets	3
Emprazil-C Tablets	5
Endep	13, 28
Enduron Tablets	24
Enduronyl Forte Tablets	25
Enduronyl Tablets	25
Equagesic	3
Equanil	16, 19
Esgic	1
Esidrix	24
Esimil	25
Eskalith	16
Eta-Lent	22, 27
Etrafon Tablets	13, 16
Eutonyl	24
Eutroa Filmtab Tablets	25
Excedrin P.M.	1
Exna Tablets	25
Exna-R Tablets	25
Fastin Capsules	9
Fiogesic Tablets	3
Fiorinal	3
Fiorinal with Codeine	5
Gaysal	1
Gaysal S	1
Gemonil	12
Ger-O-Foam	4
Gustase-Plus	18
Harmonyl	24
Heparin Sodium	11

continued

Drug Names	Classification Number
Historal	10
Hyalex	7
Hycodan	15
Hycotuss	15
HydroDIURIL	24
Hydromox Tablets	25
Hydromox-R Tablets	25
Hydropres	25
Hygroton	24
Impramine	28, 13
Inderal	23, 24, 29
Inderide	24
Innovar Injection	5
Intal	10
INV 4-5	28, 13
Ionamin	9
Ismelin	24
Iso-Bid Capsules	27
Isordil	27
Janimine	28
LaBid 250	10
Lanoxin	26
Levo-Dromoran Injectable	5
Levo-Dromoran Tablets	5
Levsin	18
Levsinex	18
Libritabs Tablets	16
Librium	16
Lidone Capsules	16
Limbitrol Tablets	13, 16
Lioresal	20
Lipo-Hepin	11
Liquamar	11
Lithane	16
Lithium	16
Lithonate	16
Lithotabs	16
Lodiomil	28
Loniten Tablets	24
Lopressor Tablets	24
Loxitane	16
Loxitane C	16

continued

Drug Names	Classification Number
Loxitane Capsules	16
Magan	7
Maprotiline	28
Marplan Tablets	13
Maxigesic Capsules	1
Mebaral	12, 18
Mellaril	16
Menrium	16
Mepergan	19
Mepergan Injection	5
Meprospan	16
Mesantoin	12
Metahydrin	24
Metatensin	25
Metubine	20
Mianserin	28
Micrainin	16
Micronefrin	10
Midol	3
Midrin Capsules	1
Migralam Capsules	1
Milontin Kapseals and Suspension	12
Milpath	16
Milprem	16
Miltown	16
Miltrate	16
Minipress	24
Minizide Capsules	24
Minotal Tablets	1
Miradon	11
Moban	16
Mobidin	7
Moderil	24
Motrin Tablets	7
Mudrane	10
Mudrane 66	10
Mysoline	12
Nadolol	29
Nagua Tablets	24
Naloxazine	28
Naquival Tablets	25

continued

Drug Names	Classification Number
Nardil	13
Naturetin Tablets	24
Navane Capsules and Concentrate	16
Nembutal	18
Neothylline	10
Nitro-Bid	27
Nitroglyn	27
Nitrol Ointment	27
Nitrong Ointment	27
Nitrospan	27
Noctec	19
Noludar and Noludar 300	19
Norflex	20
Norgesic and Norgesic Forte	3
Norisodrine Aerotrol	10
Norpace	23
Norpramin	13, 28
Nortriptyline	28
Nubain	6
Numorphan	5
Obestat Long Acting Capsules	9
Obetrol	8
Oreticyl	25
Orinase Tablets	14
Os-Cal-Gesic Tablets	4
PMB 200 and PMB 400	16
Pabalate-SF Tablets	7
Pabalate Tablets	7
Pabirin Buffered Tablets	3
Pacaps	3
Pamelor	13, 28
Panheprin	11
Panitol Tablets	1
Pantopon	5
Panwarfarin	11
Paradione	12
Paraflex	20
Parafon Forte Tablets	1, 21
Parnate	13
Pathibamate	16
Pavabid	27

continued

Drug Names	Classification Number
Pavulon	20
Pediacof	15
Peganone	12
Pentothal	18
Pentritol-60 mg	27
Percocet	1
Percocet-5	5
Percodan and Percodan-Demi Tablets	5
Percogesic with Codeine	1, 5
Peritrate	27
Permitil Chronotab Tables, Oral Concentrate	16
Presamine	28
Persistin	3
Pertofrane	13, 28
Phenaphen with Codeine Capsules	1, 5
Phenaphen with Codeine Tablets	5
Phenergan	15, 19
Phenprocoumon	11
Phenurone	12
Phrenilin Tablets	1
Plegine	9
Plexonal	18
Pondimin Tablets	9
Ponstel	6
Prelu-2 Timed Release Capsules	9
Preludin	9
Pretts Tablets	9
Procainamide Hydrochloride	23
Procan SR	23
Prolamine Capsules	9
Prolixin	16
Pronestyl Capsules and Tabs	23
Propranolol	29
Protamine Sulfate	11
Protriptyline	28
Quaalude	19
Quibron bidCaps	10
Quide	16
Quinaglute	17, 23
Quinamm	20
Quinidex	17, 23
Quinidine	17, 23

continued

Drug Names	Classification Number
Quinidine Sulfate	23, 17
Quinite Tablets	20
Quinora	23
Raudixin Tablets	16, 24
Rau-Sed	16, 24
Rauzide	25
Remsed Tablets	19
Renese-R	25
Repan	1, 18
Rhinex D Lay	1
Robaxin	20
Robaxisal Tablets	21
Robitussin A-C	15
Ryna-CX Liquid	15
SPRX-105 Capsules	9
S-T Forte Syrup and Sugar-Free	15
Saluron	24
Salutensin/Salutensin-Demi	25
Sanorex	9
Sarapin	7
Seconal Sodium	18
Sedapap 10	18, 1
Ser-Ap-Es	25
Serax	16
Serentil	16
Serpasil	16, 24
Serpasil-Apresoline	24
Serpasil-Esidrix	25
Sinequan	16, 28
Singlet	1
Sinubid	1
Sinulin Tablets	1
Sintrom	11
Sio-Phyllin Gyrocaps, Tablets	10
SK-Pramine	28
Skelaxin Tablets	20
Solfoton	18
Soma	20, 21
Sorbitrate Tablets	27
Spironolactone with Hydrochlorothiazide Tablets	24
Stadol	6
Statobex	9

continued

Drug Names	Classification Number
Statobex-G Tablets	9
Stelazine	16
Sublimaze Injection	5
Sucostrin Injection, for Infusion, High Potency	20
Supac	3
Surmontil	13, 28
Sus-Phrine	10
Synalgos Capsules	3
Synalgos-DC Capsules	5
Synophylate	10
Talwin Compound	6
Talwin 50	6
Talwin Injection	6
Taractan	16
Tegretol	6, 12
Tenormin	29
Tenuate Dospan	9
Tepanil	9
Theo-Dur Tablets	10
Theobid, Theobid Jr. Duracap	10
Theoclear	10, 22, 27
Theophyl Chewable Tablets	10
Theolair	10
Theovent Long-Acting Capsules	10
Thorazine	16
Tofranil	13, 28
Timolol	29
Tolbutamide Tablets	14
Tolinase Tablets	14
Trancopal	16
Tranxene	16
Triavil	16
Tridione	12
Trilafon	16
Trimipramine	28
Tubucurarine Chloride	20
Tuinal	18
Tussar	15
Tussend Expectorant	15
Tussi-Organdin	15
Tussionex Tablets, Capsules and Suspension	15

continued

Drug Names	Classification Number
Tylenol	1
Tylenol with Codeine Elixir	5
Tylenol with Codeine Tablets	5
Tylox Capsules	5
Unisome	19
Urispas	22
Unitensen	24
Valium	12, 16, 20
Vanceril Inhaler	10
Vanquish	3
Vasospan	27
Vesprin	16
Vicodin	5
Vistaril	16
Vivactyl	13, 28
Voranil	9
Warfarin	11
Wygesic Tablets	6
Zarontin Capsules and Syrup	12
Zaroxolyn	24
Zimelidine	28
Zomax Tablets	8

Review dispatch information
- Route
- Anticipate type of problems

Overview the scene
- Hazards, guns, crowd, gas, electric
- Exit routes, position of patients
- Cause of injuries

Protect the neck

Treat

- Airway
  - Insure continued airway/assist respiration
- Bleeding
  - Control major bleeding first
- Circulation
  - CPR
  - Start shock treatment, if indicated

HEAD-TO-TOE

VITAL SIGNS

Pulse

- Rate ________
  - Adult 60-80
  - Ped 80-100
  - Infant 120-160
- Rhythm
  - regular
  - irregular
- Quality
  - weak
  - thready
  - normal
  - pounding

Respirations

- Rate ________
  - Adult 16-20
  - Ped 20-28
  - Infant 28-36
- Rhythm
  - regular
  - Biots
  - Cheyne-Stokes
  - Kussmaul

continued

- Depth
  - deep
  - normal
  - shallow
- Odors
  - blood
  - vomit
  - acetone
  - alcohol
- Sputum
  - red blood
  - pink, frothy
  - green, yellow, gray sooty
- Sounds
  - wheezes
  - rales
  - ronchi
  - stridor
- Labored
  - normal
  - mild
  - retraction (marked)

Bp ______ / ______

Orthostatic changes

______ / ______ → P ______

______ / ______ ↑ P ______

Skin

- Temp
  - cool
  - warm (98.6F 37C)
  - hot
- Moisture
  - dry
  - moist
  - sweaty
- Color
  - pink
  - red
  - pale (pallor)
  - blue (cyanosis)
  - gray (ashen)
  - yellow (jaundice)

---

continued

Pupils	• PERLA (pupils equal & react to light/accomodating) • constricted • dialated • fixed • unequal (R larger, L larger) • unreactive (R, L) • wandering • gaze
Level of consciousness	• Loss of consciousness - yes - lucid interval • CAO - person - place - time • Lethargic • Coma - verbal - noxious - postures - inappropriate - appropriate - no response • Sensation - all extremities • Motion - all extremities • Reflexes - equal - unequal - clonus - Babinski

PHYSICAL EXAM

All body parts will be checked for: open wounds, deformities, swelling, bruising and pain (lesions).

Head	• lesions • battle sign

continued

Eyes	• vision - normal - blurred - light only • one eye only (R, L) - normal - injury • penetrating wounds • Raccoon eyes • lesions • range of occular motion
Ears	• blood • CSF • lesions
Nose	• blood • CSF • lesions
Mouth	• teeth intact • foreign fluids • lesions
Neck	• distended veins • tracheal trauma • sub-Q air • hoarseness • lesions
Chest	• semetry/integrity • sub-Q air • breath sounds • EKG (BBB in trauma) • retraction • lesions
Back	• spine • ribs • lesions
Abdomen	• nausea and vomiting • distension • guarding • lesions • radiating pain

continued

Pelvis	• increased pain on compression • lesions • genital injuries
Limbs	• range of motion • lesions • sensation - numbness - normal - no

HISTORY

Medic-Alert	
Chief complaint	
Onset of symptoms	
Pain	• type • location • radiates to • duration • aggrevating/alleviating
Other symptoms	
Diets/medications	• last taken • dosage • allergies
Recent health	
Recent illness	
Surgeries	
Female	• last period • birth control • gestation/previous preg. • bleeding - rate - number pads used
Name	
Age/DOB	
Dr.	

PHONE NUMBERS

HOSPITALS

AMBULANCE

FIRE DEPT.

LAW

OTHERS

POISON CONTROL

HOT LINES

RADIO-TELEMETRY PHONE BOOK

Name	Radio	Channel	Channel Guard	Code Numbers/ Code Name
1.				
2.				
3.				
4.				
5.				
6.				
7.				
8.				
9.				
10.				
11.				
12.				
13.				
14.				
15.				
16.				
17.				
18.				
19.				
20.				
21.				
22.				

Bibliography

Abbott, J. et al. Protocols for prehospital emergency medical care. Baltimore: Williams and Wilkins, 1980.

Backer, C. Physician's desk reference 36. Oradell, New Jersey: Medical Economics Co., 1982.

Barber, J. M. Handbook of emergency pharmacology. St. Louis: C.V. Mosby Co., 1978.

Barber, J. and S. Budassi. Mosby's manual of emergency care. St. Louis: C.V. Mosby Co., 1979.

Cain, H. D. and T. Flint. Emergency treatment and management, ed. 5. Philadelphia: W. B. Saunders Co., 1975.

"EMT-advanced," republication edition. Department of Transportation HS 501207.

Freitag, J. and L. Miller. Manual of medical therapeutics, ed. 23. Boston: Little, Brown and Co., 1980.

Krupp, M. and M. Chatton. Current medical diagnosis and treatment 1980. Los Altos, California: Lange Medical Publications, 1980.

Luckmann, J. and K. Sorensen. Medical-surgical nursing, a psychophysiological approach. Philadelphia: W. B. Saunders Co., 1974.

Margolis, S. and J. Wasserberger. Pharmacology and therapeutics in emergency care. Denver: Multi-Media Publishing, Inc., 1982.

McIntyre, K. and A. Lewis. Textbook of advanced cardiac life support. Dallas: American Heart Association Office of Communications, 1981.

Pascoe, D. and M. Grossman. Quick reference to pediatric emergencies. Philadelphia: J. B. Lippincott Co., 1973.

Waring, W. and L. Jeansomme. Practical manual of pediatrics: a pocket reference for those who treat children. St. Louis: C. V. Mosby Co., 1975.